Viva Tutorials for Surgeons in Training

Viva Tutorials for Surgeons in Training

Editor

Reuben Johnson

Authors

Reuben Johnson
Wendy Adams
Jonathan Bull
Jonathan Epstein
Anant Krishnan
Leon Menezes
Bijan Modarai
Paul Patterson
Arun Sahai
Alexis Schizas

2004

Greenwich Medical Media Ltd

© 2004

ISBN 1841102156

First Published 2004

The publisher makes no representation, express or implied, with regard to the accuracy of the information contained in this book and cannot accept any legal responsibility or liability for any errors or omissions that may be made.

A catalogue record for this book is available from the British Library.

Typeset by Charon Tec Pvt. Ltd, Chennai, India
Printed and bound in the UK by Cambridge University Press

Contents

Authors

Reuben Johnson
BSc, MB ChB, MRCS Glasg., MRCS Eng.
Neurosurgery
Anatomy and Human Genetics
University of Oxford
Oxford

Wendy Adams
MB ChB, MRCP (UK), MRCOphth.
Ophthalmology
Northern Region SpR Rotation
Royal Victoria Infirmary
Newcastle

Jonathan Bull
MA, MB BChir, MRCS Glasg.
Neurosurgery
St Mary's/Imperial College BST
London

Jonathan Epstein
MA, BM BCh, MRCS Eng.
General Surgery and Critical Care
Christie Hospital
Manchester

Anant Krishnan
BSc, MB BS, MRCS Eng.
Neuroradiology and Molecular Imaging
University of Cambridge
Cambridge

Leon Menezes
MA, BM BCh, MRCP
Radiology
Guy's and St Thomas' Hospitals
London

Bijan Modarai
BSc, MB BS, MRCS Ed., MRCS Eng.
Vascular Surgery
Guy's and St Thomas' Hospitals
London

Paul Patterson
MB BS, FRCS Ed.
Trauma and Orthopaedics
Northern Region SpR Rotation,
North Tyneside General Hospital
Newcastle

Arun Sahai
BSc, MB BS, MRCS Eng.
Urology
Guy's and St Thomas' Hospitals
London

Alexis Schizas
BSc, MB BS, MRCS Eng.
General Surgery
Guy's and St Thomas' Hospitals
London

Preface

This volume has been designed specifically for candidates preparing for the MRCS Viva. The viva format of the examination has been used with over *1000 questions* to illustrate the key points of over *200 topics*. The book has been divided into six sections, each one corresponding to a viva station in the examination. The individual sections begin with a checklist and take the reader logically and systematically through the main topics and themes covered by the examination. Key concepts are covered in all areas and in some cases topics are covered in more detail than would be asked in the examination. The candidate using this book for viva practice in their revision schedule should be able to enter the examination room with confidence.

Reuben Johnson
Oxford, 2004

Applied Surgical Anatomy

SECTION

1

HEAD AND NECK

THORAX

ABDOMEN AND PELVIS

Applied Surgical Anatomy

LIMBS

1. Fascial Compartments of the Neck

What is the significance of the fascial compartments of the neck?
They compartmentalise structures in the neck and form natural planes of cleavage through which tissues can be separated in surgery. They also form planes along which infections can spread.

What are the different fascial layers?
They are made up of superficial and deep cervical fascia. Superficial fascia lies between the skin and investing layer of deep fascia. As well as containing nerves, blood vessels and lymphatics, it encloses the platysma muscle anteriorly. The deep cervical fascia consists of four parts: investing; pretracheal; prevertebral; and the carotid sheath.

Can you tell me the margins of the investing layer?
The investing layer of fascia surrounds the neck deep to the superficial fascial layer. It splits to enclose the trapezius and sternocleidomastoid muscles on either side. The superior attachment of the investing layer extends from the superior nuchal line to the tip of the mastoid process. It extends to the zygomatic arch and the lower border of the mandible. Anteriorly, it attaches to the hyoid bone and posteriorly, it attaches to the ligamentum nuchae. Between the angle of the mandible and mastoid process, it splits to enclose the parotid and submandibular glands. Inferiorly, it attaches to the manubrium, clavicles and the spines and acromion of the scapulae. In attaching to the manubrium, the investing layer attaches to the anterior and posterior border forming a suprasternal space.

Can you do the same for the pretracheal fascia?
The pretracheal fascia lies deep to the strap muscles of the neck. It extends from its superior attachment, the hyoid bone, down to merge with the fibrous pericardium and adventitia of the arch of the aorta. It splits to enclose the thyroid gland, trachea and oesophagus and blends laterally with the carotid sheath.

And the prevertebral fascia?
The prevertebral fascia lies in front of the prevertebral muscles. It extends from the base of the skull to the body of the third thoracic vertebra. It extends to the side covering the muscles of the floor of the posterior triangle. The cervical and brachial plexi lie deep. The

prevertebral fascia extends laterally to cover the subclavian artery and continues under the clavicle as the axillary sheath.

Where does the carotid sheath run?

The carotid sheath surrounds the carotid arteries, internal jugular vein and vagus nerve. It is a tubular attachment extending from the base of the skull to the root of the neck.

Why is it clinically important to understand the fascial planes?

The fascial compartments limit the spread of infection to within that fascial plane. For example, an infection within the investing layer limits infection to the superior margin of the manubrium. However, infection may spread within the spaces between the fascial compartments. The most important of these spaces are the prevertebral, retropharyngeal, parapharyngeal and submandibular spaces.

Can you tell me more about these spaces and the effect of infection here?

Infection between the investing and pretracheal layers can lead to infection spreading to the thoracic cavity. The retropharyngeal space lies between the prevertebral fascia and the fascia covering the pharnx. A retropharyngeal abscess may result in oedema and dysphagia. The submandibular space extends above the investing layer of fascia to the floor of the mouth. Infection in this space can lead to cellulitis – Ludwig's Angina. The prevertebral space is closed behind the prevertebral fascia and an abscess there can extend as low as the third thoracic vertebra.

2. Posterior Triangle of the Neck

What are the boundaries of the posterior triangle?
- Anteriorly: the posterior border of sternocleidomastoid.
- Posteriorly: the anterior border of trapezius.
- Inferiorly: the middle third of the clavicle.

The apex of the triangle is on the back of the skull on the superior nuchal line. The roof is formed by the investing layer of deep cervical fascia. The floor is formed by the prevertebral fascia.

What layers would you go through making an incision here?

An incision into the posterior triangle passes through skin, subcutaneous fat, platysma, investing layer of deep cervical fascia to enter the posterior triangle.

What muscles lie beneath the prevertebral fascia?

From superolateral to inferomedial:

- splenius capitis,
- levator scapulae,
- scalenus posterior,
- scalenus medius,
- scalenus anterior.

Are you able to further subdivide the posterior triangle?

The omohyoid muscle divides the posterior triangle into the supraclavicular triangle inferiorly and the occipital triangle superiorly.

What are the contents of the posterior triangle?

The contents of the posterior triangle can be divided into arteries, veins, nerves and lymphatics.

- Arteries: third part of subclavian artery, transverse cervical artery, suprascapular artery and occipital artery.
- Veins: external jugular vein, subclavian vein, transverse cervical vein, suprascapular vein and anterior jugular veins.
- Nerves: Spinal accessory nerve, posterior branch of cervical plexus and the trunks of brachial plexus.
- Lymph nodes: cervical lymph nodes and supraclavicular lymph nodes.

Can you tell me the surface marking of the spinal accessory nerve?

The surface marking of the spinal accessory nerve in the posterior triangle follows a line originating at the junction of the superior one-third to inferior two-thirds of the sternocleidomastoid muscle extending to a point on the anterior border of trapezius 5 cm above the clavicle.

What would the clinical effect be of cutting the spinal accessory nerve in the posterior triangle?

Injury to the spinal accessory nerve leads to an inability to shrug the shoulder and abduct the arm above 90 degrees.

3. Thyroid Gland

How does the thyroid gland develop?

The thyroid gland develops in the floor of the mouth and migrates inferiorly. It passes from the foramen caecum through the thyroglossal duct via hyoid bone to its usual position in the neck.

What is the position of the thyroid gland in the neck?

The two lobes of the thyroid lie lateral to the trachea and are connected by an isthmus which is attached to the second to fourth tracheal rings. It is enclosed by pretracheal fascia, which also attaches the thyroid to the trachea at this point. This is why the thyroid moves up with the larynx during swallowing.

What are the relations of the thyroid gland?

- Anterolaterally: strap muscles (sternothyroid and sternohyoid).
- Posteriorly: carotid sheaths and parathyroid glands.
- Medially: upper trachea, larynx, oesophagus, pharynx, inferior constrictor, cricothyroid, external laryngeal nerves and recurrent laryngeal nerves.

What layers would you go through to access the thyroid gland?

The layers exposed to access the thyroid gland are skin, subcutaneous fat, platysma, investing layer of deep cervical fascia, strap muscles (sternothyroid and sternohyoid) and pretracheal fascia.

What is the arterial supply of the thyroid gland?

- Superior thyroid artery: first branch of external carotid artery (at the superior pole of the gland, the external laryngeal nerve lies behind the artery).
- Inferior thyroid artery: thyrocervical trunk (the recurrent laryngeal nerve has a variable relationship with the inferior thyroid artery).
- Thyroidea ima artery: occasionally present from the brachiocephalic trunk or arch of the aorta.

What is the venous drainage of the thyroid gland?

- Superior thyroid veins (into the internal jugular veins).
- Middle thyroid veins (into the internal jugular veins).
- Inferior thyroid veins (into the brachiocephalic veins).

What is the effect of damage to the recurrent laryngeal nerve?

- Unilateral damage to the recurrent laryngeal nerve can lead to a hoarse voice.
- Bilateral damage leads to complete cord paralysis and requires the insertion of a tracheostomy.

What is the effect of damage to the external laryngeal nerve?

Damage to the external laryngeal nerve leads to a voice that is monotonous in character due to paralysis of the cricothyroid muscle.

Where are the parathyroid glands situated?

There are four parathyroid glands which usually lie behind the thyroid gland. The upper glands are fourth branchial arch derivatives whereas the lower glands are third branchial arch derivatives. These glands are occasionally found in the mediastinum. All the glands are supplied by the inferior thyroid artery. It is of note that the parathyroid gland was first discovered in a rhinoceros by Richard Owen who performed a post-mortem on the animal to determine the cause of death while it was in captivity at London Zoo. The dissected rhinoceros larynx is still on display in the Hunterian museum of the Royal College of Surgeons of London.

4. Parotid Gland

Describe the position of the parotid gland without touching your face.

The parotid gland sits between the styloid and mastoid processes of the temporal bone and the ramus of the mandible and runs out over these bones.

What type of gland is the parotid?

A serous salivary gland.

What nerve lies within the substance of the gland? Describe its course.

The facial nerve (VIIth cranial nerve). The facial nerve emerges from the skull base through the stylomastoid foramen and passes into the posterior surface of the parotid gland. It bifurcates into upper and lower divisions. The upper division gives rise to the temporal and zygomatic branches, the lower to buccal, marginal mandibular and cervical branches. All these branches leave the gland through its anterior surface. Connections exist between the branches within the substance of the gland but injury to these connections at surgery is rarely significant.

How does the facial nerve come to lie within the parotid gland?

The parotid gland develops in the "V" between the upper and lower divisions of the facial nerve but as it develops it comes to engulf and surround the nerve.

Aside from injury to the facial nerve what other specific complications can arise from parotidectomy?
Injury to the greater auricular nerve can lead to loss of sensation to the earlobe (making it difficult to wear ear-rings).

Frey's syndrome – gustatory sweating, thought to result from cross-over between sympathetic and parasympathetic fibres.

5. Submandibular Region

Which muscles in the submandibular region are developed from the first pharyngeal arch?
Mylohyoid and the anterior belly of digastric which are both supplied by the V nerve.

Which muscles in the submandibular region are developed from the second pharyngeal arch?
Stylohyoid and the posterior belly of digastric which are both supplied by the VIIth cranial nerve.

What is the relation of the submandibular gland and submandibular duct to mylohoid?
The submandibular gland is a "U"-shaped gland which arches around the posterior extremity of mylohyoid: it is, therefore, both superficial and deep to mylohyoid. The submandibular duct lies deep to mylohyoid.

What is the relationship of the sublingual gland to mylohyoid?
The gland lies superficial to mylohyoid.

What is the relationship of the lingual nerve and the lingual artery to the hyoglossus muscle?
The lingual nerve runs superficial, or lateral, to the hyoglossus whereas the lingual artery runs deep, or medial, to the hyoglossus.

What is the relation of the lingual nerve to the submandibular duct?
Initially, the lingual nerve runs lateral to the duct but then it loops underneath it to run medial to it into the tongue.

6. Pharynx

What is the pharynx?

The pharynx is essentially a musculofascial tube which extends from the base of the skull to the oesophagus and larynx (C6 level): it is a common entrance to the respiratory tract (via larynx) and the alimentary tract (via oesophagus).

What are the layers of the pharynx?

The four layers of the pharynx are, from innermost out:

1. mucous membrane,
2. submucusa,
3. muscular layer,
4. buccopharyngeal membrane.

How is the muscular organised?

The muscles of the pharynx are organised into an outer group of constrictors (superior, middle and inferior constrictors) and an inner group of longitudinal muscles (palatopharyngeus, stylopharyngeus and salpingopharyngeus).

What is Killian's dehiscence?

The inferior constrictor muscle actually consists of two parts: thyropharyngeus and cricopharyngeus. There is a small gap between the two known as Killian's dehiscence through which the mucosa may protrude to form a pharyngeal pouch.

What are the three regions of the pharynx?

The nasopharynx, the oropharynx and the laryngopharynx.

Can you name two important anatomical structures in the nasopharynx?

- The nasopharyngeal tonsils (adenoids) which are prominent in children.
- The orifice of the Eustachian tube.

What muscles form the anterior and posterior pillars in the oropharynx?

- Anterior pillar: palatoglossus.
- Posterior pillar: palatopharyngeus.

Where in the pharynx are the palatine tonsils located and what is their arterial supply?

The palatine tonsil is located in the oropharynx between the anterior and posterior pillars. The arterial supply is via tonsilar branch of the facial artery.

What is the name given to the ring of lymphoid tissue that surrounds the pharynx?

Waldeyer's ring.

What is the nerve supply to the pharynx?

All muscles are supplied by the pharyngeal plexus (IX and X) except cricopharyngeus which is supplied by the external laryngeal nerve. Sensation to the nasopharynx is supplied by the maxillary branch of V and to the oropharynx by the IXth cranial nerve.

7. Larynx

What is the function of the larynx?

The primary function of the larynx is to protect the airway from inhalation of foreign bodies. It also has a secondary function in phonation.

What types of structures make up the larynx?

The larynx is a framework of articulating cartilages linked by ligaments.

Can you name the cartilaginous parts of the larynx and do you know at which vertebral levels they are found?

Although not strictly cartilaginous, the hyoid bone lies superiorly at the C3 level. Below the hyoid bone is the thyroid cartilage with its upper limit at C4 and the cricoid cartilage at C6. The epiglottis is a large cartilaginous structure within the larynx which reaches as high as C3. The arytenoids cartilages lie within the larynx at the C5 level. The corniculate and cuneiform cartilages are also found in the larynx?

What are the pharyngeal arch derivatives of the hyoid bone, thyroid cartilage and cricoid cartilage?

The body of the hyoid lies at C3 and is a third arch derivative. The thyroid cartilage lies at C4 and is a fourth arch derivative. The cricoid lies at C6 and is a sixth arch derivative.

Can you name the extrinsic ligaments of the larynx?

There are four main extrinsic ligaments in the larynx:

- thyrohyoid ligament,
- hyoepiglottic ligament,
- cricotracheal ligament,
- cricothyroid ligament.

What is the conus elastica?

The conus elastica is the tent-like cricovocal membrane. Thickening of this structure gives rise to the cricothyroid ligament anteriorly and the vocal cords superiorly.

Can you describe the spaces in and around the larynx?

Either side of the epiglottis is the *piriform fossa* which is bordered by the lower pharynx on either side. The inlet of the larynx, or *aditus*, is formed by the upper lip of the epiglottis anteriorly and anterolaterally, the aryepiglottic folds posterolaterally, and the transverse interarytenoid fold posteriorly. The *vestibule* of the larynx is the supraglottic compartment of the larynx between the aditus and false cords. The *glottis* lies between the vestibular folds and the rima glottidis. Within the glottis are bilateral *laryngeal sinuses* and *laryngeal saccules* formed by folds of mucosa.

Which nerve supplies the extrinsic muscles of the larynx?

Cranial nerve XII.

Which muscles hold the vocal cords open and what is the nerve supply?

The posterior cricoarytenoids hold the vocal cords open by externally rotating the arytenoids. They are supplied by the recurrent laryngeal nerve.

8. Infratemporal Fossa

What are the boundaries of the infratemporal fossa?

- Superiorly: the temporal bone and the greater wing of the sphenoid.
- Anteriorly: the posterior surface of the maxilla.
- Medially: the lateral pterygoid plate.
- Laterally: the ramus of the mandible.
- Posteriorly: the carotid sheath.
- Inferiorly: free.

What are the important contents of the infratemporal fossa?

- Maxillary artery.
- Mandibular nerve.
- Medial and lateral pterygoid muscles.
- Otic ganglion.

- Chorda tympani.
- Pterygoid venous plexus.
- Posterior superior alveolar nerve.

How many branches does the maxillary artery have?

The maxillary artery have 15 branches.

Which of these branches is the most important to clinically?

The middle meningeal artery, the rupture of which is a common cause of extradural haematoma.

How does this artery enter the skull?

It passes through the foramen spinosum.

9. Surface Anatomy of Thorax

What is the angle of Louis?
The angle of Louis is the transverse ridge of the manubriosternal joint.

What is the significance of the angle of Louis?
It is at the level of the second costal cartilage making it possible to accurately map out the second intercostal space. This space is used (in the midclavicular line) for emergency decompression of a tension pneumothorax. In addition, it provides a point from which to accurately and count down to the other ribs, e.g., to find the appropriate site to insert an intercostal drain (fifth intercostal space in the anterior axillary line).

The angle of Louis also lies at the level of the intervertebral disc between the fourth and fifth thoracic vertebrae. This level corresponds to:

- the bifurcation of the trachea into the two major bronchi,
- the entry of the azygous vein into the superior vena cava,
- the start and finish of the arch of the aorta.

Can you mark out the surface anatomy of the pleura?
Beginning at the sternoclavicular joint the pleural reflection passes behind this structure and descends to meet in the midline at the angle of Louis. On the right it passes down in a curved manner behind the sternum to the sixth costal cartilage, and then to the eighth rib in the midclavicular line, tenth rib in the midaxillary line and twelfth rib at the lateral border of erector spinae. It is noteworthy that the pleura extends just below the twelfth rib at its medial aspect – a point well remembered by urologists in their posterior approach to the kidney. On the left, the pleura descends initially until the fourth costal cartilage where it arches to the left to accommodate the pericardium and from here descends lateral to the sternum. Otherwise, the relations of the pleura are the same on either side. Above the sternoclavicular joint the pleurae ascend above the clavicle for about 2.5 cm and this point corresponds to the apex of the pleura.

Can you describe some surface markings to outline the heart?
The apex beat, in a health adult, lies in the midclavicular line at the level of the fifth intercostal space. This corresponds to the left lower extremity of the heart. The right lower extremity is surface marked by

the sixth costal cartilage, half an inch from the sternal edge. The third costal cartilage on the right and the second on the left mark the upper extremities, both half an inch from their respective sides of the sternal edge.

What are your landmarks for needle insertion and direction in emergency pericardiocentesis?

When performing pericardiocentesis in an emergency situation, the surgeon should place the needle 1–2 cm below and to the left of the xiphoid and advance the needle at an angle of 45 degrees in the direction of the tip of the left scapula.

How could you accurately mark out the oblique and transverse fissures of the lung?

The oblique fissure, which divides the lungs into upper and lower borders, can be represented by fully abducting the shoulder. The line of the oblique fissure corresponds to the medial border of the scapula. Alternatively, this can be marked by a line joining a point 1 inch lateral from the spine of the fifth thoracic vertebra in an oblique downward and outward fashion to meet the sixth costal cartilage. The transverse fissure separates the middle and upper lobes of the right lung. Its surface marking is a line drawn horizontally along the fourth costal cartilage, meeting the oblique fissure as it crosses the fifth rib.

At what vertebral level does the trachea commence and can this level be surface marked?

The trachea begins at the level of C6, this corresponds to the lower border of the cricoid cartilage. As discussed previously, the trachea descends vertically downwards and ends at the level of T4/T5, at the level of the angle of Louis.

10. Thoracic Vertebra

What are the typical components of a vertebra?

A classical vertebra is made up of a body and neural arch. The neural arch surrounds the vertebral canal and arises from the posterior aspect of the body. The arch consists of a pedicle on either side, which on its inferior and superior aspects forms a notch. When the vertebrae are aligned these notches (an inferior notch of one vertebra and the superior pedicle notch of the vertebra below) form the intervertebral foramen. Segmental spinal nerves are carried within the foramen. The rest of the arch is formed by paired lamina, again one on either side, which can be thought of as a continuation of the pedicles. The laminae join in the midline posteriorly and from this point the spine of the vertebra arises. In addition, the arch conveys two lateral transverse processes (these processes act as a landmark separating pedicles from laminae) and superior and inferior facets for articulation with vertebrae above and below.

How do thoracic vertebrae differ from other vertebrae?

Thoracic vertebrae harbour facets on the side of their bodies and on their transverse processes for articulation with ribs. This fact makes distinguishing them beyond doubt if asked to pick one up from a box full of different vertebrae in the viva. Other clues to distinguish them quickly are that in general their spinous processes tend to be longer and slope downwards when compared to others.

What layers would an anaesthetist go through in placing a thoracic epidural?

The layers traversed would be:

- skin,
- subcutaneous fat,
- deep fascia,
- supraspinous ligaments,
- interspinous ligaments,
- extradural fat (containing the venous plexus).

If you feel a give then it is likely that the needle has penetrated the dura, and potentially entered the subarachnoid space (this is confirmed by the aspiration of cerebrospinal fluid, CSF).

At what level do thoracic vertebral fractures most commonly occur and why?

T-spine fractures are common at the thoraco-lumbar junction. Although there is relatively little movement between vertebrae this is exaggerated at the cervico-thoracic and particularly at the thoraco-lumbar junctions. Classically the injury is a flexion/compression injury.

11. Ribs

What is the difference between true and false ribs?

True ribs, 1–7, are directly attached to the sternum via their own costal cartilage. False ribs, 8–10, have their costal cartilage attach to the cartilage of the rib above, and are not directly attached to the sternum. Ribs 11 and 12 do not attach to the sternum and are therefore sometimes called floating ribs.

Describe a typical rib.

A typical rib bears two facets on its head for articulation with the corresponding vertebra and the vertebra above. It has a neck and a tubercle which also articulates with the transverse process of the corresponding vertebra. The rest of the rib is made up of the shaft. The ribs are angled downward and curve in a semicircular fashion anteriorly to attach the sternum via costal cartilages. The point at which the shaft curves the most is known as the angle and the inner aspect of the rib is lined by the subcostal groove.

What is different about the first rib?

The first rib is the shortest, flattest and most curved of all the ribs. It is an atypical rib in that it has only one facet at its head for articulation with its corresponding vertebral body. In addition, it displays the scalene tubercle on its upper surface and posterior to this lies the subclavian groove.

What can you tell me about the scalene tubercle and its surrounding structures?

Scalenus anterior, arising from the cervical vertebrae, attaches the scalene tubercle. The subclavian groove, which lies just posterior to the tubercle is occupied by the lowest trunk of the brachial plexus and is related intimately to the second part of the subclavian artery. Anterior to the scalene tubercle runs the subclavian vein in its own groove.

What structures are directly anterior to the first rib?

Three structures lie anterior to the neck of the first rib. These are, from medial to lateral: the sympathetic trunk (stellate ganglion), the superior intercostal arteryand the first thoracic nerve.

What do you know about cervical ribs and their presentation?

A cervical rib occurs in approximately 0.5% of the population, and of these 50% are bilateral. It is a bony or fibrous extra rib at the level of C7. It usually articulates with the first rib but may be free. The problem with this extra rib is that it may contribute to thoracic outlet syndrome (70% are asymptomatic). This is a condition with various aetiologies of which one is cervical rib, leads to the impingement of neurovascular structures at the root of the neck. The patient may present with symptoms related to impingement of the lowest trunk of the brachial plexus. Thus the resultant pain and paraesthesia will be in the distribution of the ulnar nerve. Classically, the patient presents with wasting of the muscles of the hand (T1). If there is impingement of the subclavian artery, symptoms related to post-stenotic dilatation and thrombus formation may occur. This has a varied spectrum from intermittent claudication in the affected limb to frank gangrene. If the history it is at all suspicious a chest X-ray (CXR) must be carried out to exclude the possibility of a cervical rib.

12. Intercostal Space

What are the contents of the intercostal space?
The space contains three muscles and a neurovascular bundle. The muscles from outside-in are the external intercostal, the internal intercostal and the innermost intercostal muscle.

In what layer is the neurovascular bundle found? What is it composed of?
The neurovascular bundle lies between the inner and innermost intercostal muscles. From superior to inferior lie the intercostal vein, artery and nerve. The arteries consist of anterior and posterior branches. The anterior branches of spaces 1–6 are derived from the internal thoracic artery directly. The anterior branches of spaces 7–9 are derived from the musculophrenic artery. The tenth and eleventh intercostal spaces are only supplied by posterior intercostal arteries. The posterior intercostals are derived directly from the descending aorta at each corresponding level. The exception to this rule is that the first two spaces (1–2) which are supplied by branches from the superior intercostal artery, which is a branch of the costocervical trunk arising from the second part of the subclavian artery. The intercostal nerves are anterior primary rami of the segmental thoracic nerves which all have muscular and cutaneous branches.

What are the landmarks for insertion of a chest drain?
Fifth intercostal space in the anterior axillary line. The midaxillary line is not used for fear of damage to nerve to serratus anterior, the long thoracic nerve and the lateral thoracic artery.

What layers would your chest tube pass before entering the pleural cavity?
The following layers would be passed through:

- skin,
- subcutaneous fat,
- deep fascia,
- serratus anterior muscle,
- external intercostal muscle,
- internal intercostal muscle,

- innermost intercostal muscle,
- endothoracic fascia,
- parietal pleural membrane.

How is the risk of damage to the neurovascular bundle minimised?

By inserting the needle superior to the rib.

What incisions do you know for access to the thoracic cavity?

The two classical incisions are the median sternotomy and a lateral thoracotomy, which can be anterolateral or posterolateral. The thoraco-abdominal approach is another option.

Describe the incision and important structures you would come across in one of these approaches.

In a posterolateral approach, the incision is made from a point midway between the midline posteriorly and the medial border of the scapula, curved anteriorly to the anterior axillary line, usually in the fifth inter-costal space (this may change depending on the site of the pathology). Important structures one would come across are as follows:

- skin,
- subcutaneous fat,
- deep fascia,
- trapezius muscle,
- latissimus dorsi muscle,
- rhomboids (major and minor),
- external intercostals muscle,

- internal intercostals muscle,
- innermost intercostals muscle,
- endothoracic fascia,
- parietal pleura,
- pleural cavity,
- visceral pleura,
- lung substance.

13. Trachea

At what vertebral level does the trachea commence and terminate?

It begins at the level of C6 at the lower border of the cricoid cartilage and terminates by splitting into the two main bronchi at T4/T5.

What are its relations in the neck?

- Anteriorly: thyroid gland, pretracheal fascia, sternohyoid and sternothyroid.
- Posteriorly: recurrent laryngeal nerves and oesophagus.

- Laterally: left and right lobes of thyroid gland, carotid sheath and its contents (internal jugular vein, common carotid artery and vagus nerve).

In what circumstances would you need to perform an emergency surgical airway in a trauma patient?

In the emergency trauma situation a surgical airway is indicated if a tracheal intubation is unsuccessful or would be dangerous to perform (e.g. in severe maxillofacial trauma). In the emergency setting there will not be time to perform a formal tracheostomy. The priority is to secure an airway even if temporary, as quickly as possible.

What technique would you employ to perform an emergency surgical airway?

The technique to employ in this situation would be dependent upon the level of expertise of the surgeon. Needle cricothyroidotomy is best performed if you are not able to perform a surgical cricothyroidotomy quickly. A 12- or 14-gauge cannula is placed through the cricothyroid membrane. This is then connected via a Y-connector to an oxygen supply. Using a jet-insufflation technique (1 second on and 4 seconds off) oxygen is delivered to the patient. This is a temporary manoeuvre to save life before a formal tracheostomy is performed.

What layers are encountered in an tracheostomy?

- Skin.
- Subcutaneous fat.
- Platysma.
- Investing layer of fascia.
- Strap muscles (sternohyoid and sternothyroid).
- Pre-tracheal fascia.
- Isthmus of the thyroid gland.
- Trachea.

Can you describe an elective tracheostomy?

This procedure can be performed under local or general anaesthesia with the patient in the supine position and the head slightly extended. An aseptic technique is employed and an injection of 1/200,000 adrenaline solution can be used for purposes of haemostasis. A horizontal incision half-way between the suprasternal notch and the cricoid cartilage. Strap muscles of the neck are divided vertically. Thyroid isthmus is divided in between two clips and secured by oversewing the edges or a secure ligature. The anterior tracheal wall is exposed. Haemostasis is achieved – this may involve ligation of inferior thyroid veins and diathermy or ligatures to the vessels supplying the strap muscles. A vertical incision centred over third to fourth tracheal rings for 2 cm. A cuffed tracheostomy tube is inserted while the incision is held open with a tracheal dilator. Inflate the cuff and connect the ventilation apparatus. Close the skin loosely around the tracheal tube. Alternatively, when the anterior trachea is exposed, some clinicians prefer to cut out an oval disc of tissue including the cartilage of the anterior wall. Ideally this should encompass the third and fourth tracheal rings. Other clinicians prefer the technique described above as they feel there is a reduced incidence of tracheal stenosis if no tissue is cut, this is particularly so if the first ring is removed.

What complications are associated with tracheostomy?

- Early: haemorrhage, tracheal/paratracheal trauma, pneumothorax, tube dislodgment, subcutaneous emphysema, infection, tube lumen obstruction with resultant apnoea and death.
- Late: difficult extubation, tracheal stenosis, tracheo-malacia, tracheo-oesophageal or tracheo-cutaneous fistulae.

14. Lungs

What are the surface markings of the lungs?

The apex of each lung is approximately 1 inch above the clavicle. The medial border of the right lung descends vertically from the second to fifth costal cartilages, near the midline. On the left, the medial border runs laterally between the fourth and fifth intercostal spaces to accommodate the heart. The lower borders of each lung slope laterally to reach the level of the sixth rib in the midclavicular line, the eighth rib at the midaxillary line and the tenth rib at the lateral border of erector spinae.

How can you locate the oblique fissure on each side?

When the arms are fully raised above the head a line represented by the vertebral border of the scapula marks out the oblique fissures.

What are the components of the left lung root?

Superiorly lies the left pulmonary artery with the left main bronchus is below it. There are two pulmonary veins: one below and one in front of the bronchus. Bronchial vessels, autonomic nerves, lymph nodes and lymphatic channels accompany these structures.

What is unusual about the blood supply to the lungs?

There is a dual supply created by anastomosis between the bronchial arteries and the pulmonary arteries.

15. Heart

What are the surface markings of the heart?

Superiorly the heart gives rise to the great vessels. The right border is formed entirely by the right atrium and extends from right third to sixth costal cartilages approximately 3 cm from the midline. The inferior border consists of right and left ventricles and runs from 3 cm to the right of the midline at the level of the sixth costal cartilage to the apex (usually fifth left intercostal space in the midclavicular line). The left border consists of left ventricle/auricle of left atrium and extends between the apex and the second left intercostal space approximately 3 cm from the midline.

How are the layers of pericardium arranged?

There are three layers of pericardium. The fibrous pericardium is the single outer layer covering the heart which fuses with the adventitia of the great vessels and is attached to the central tendon of the diaphragm. The serous pericardium lies beneath the fibrous pericardium and consists of parietal and visceral layers. The transverse and oblique sinuses form between these two layers.

Identify the main groups of veins draining the heart.

The coronary sinus is situated in the posterior atrioventricular groove and drains into the right atrium. The anterior cardiac veins open directly into the right atrium. In addition, there are numerous venae cordis minimae are small veins that drain directly into the nearest cardiac chamber.

What is the origin of the coronary arteries?

The left coronary artery originate from the left posterior aortic sinus and the right coronary artery originates from the anterior aortic sinus. These sinuses are located in the ascending aorta, just above the aortic valve.

What is a patent ductus arteriosus?

The ductus arteriosus (originating from the left sixth aortic arch) connects the pulmonary trunk to the aorta and allows blood to bypass the lungs in the foetal circulation. This connection normally closes at

Applied Surgical Anatomy

birth. A patent duct leads to shunting of blood from right to left side of the heart and pulmonary hypertension.

16. Vagus Nerve

Behind what structure does the left vagus nerve enter the chest?
The left common carotid artery.

Are the vagal nerves located in front or behind the lung roots?
Both nerves pass behind the lung roots.

How do the left and right vagus nerves terminate?
The two nerves form a plexus on the surface of the oesophagus. From this plexus anterior and posterior vagal trunks pass through the diaphragm with the oesophagus at the level of the tenth thoracic vertebra.

What is the function of the cardiac branches of the vagus nerves?
This is the parasympathetic supply to the heart. Stimulation reduces the heart rate. Loss of vagal tone causes a rise in basal heart rate.

How does the vagus contribute to pleural sensation?
Branches from the vagus provide an autonomic supply to the pleura allowing sensation to stretch.

17. Phrenic Nerve

Can you describe the origin of the phrenic nerve in the neck?
The phrenic nerves arise bilaterally from the C3, C4 and C5 nerve roots (mainly C4) and run over the anterior scalene muscles before entering the chest.

What structures do the phrenic nerves supply?
- Motor supply: muscles of the diaphragm (excluding crura).
- Sensory supply: the diaphragm, mediastinal pleura, diaphragmatic pleura, diaphragmatic peritoneum and fibrous pericardium.

Which structure does the right phrenic nerve accompany as it travels to the undersurface of the diaphragm?

It passes with the inferior vena cava through an opening in the central part of the diaphragm.

Where do you feel referred pain from the diaphragm?

In the cutaneous area representing the C4 dermatome, i.e. the shoulder tip.

What is the evidence of phrenic nerve palsy on a CXR?

Paralysis leads to elevation of the dome of the diaphragm.

18. Sympathetic Trunk

What is the course of the sympathetic trunk in the thorax?

It descends from the cervical chain along the neck of the first rib, along the heads of the second to tenth ribs, and over the bodies of the eleventh and twelfth thoracic vertebrae.

What is the stellate ganglion?

This is in fact two ganglia together: the first thoracic sympathetic ganglion joined with the inferior cervical ganglion.

How many named splanchnic nerves do you know and what are their root values?

- Greater splanchnic nerve (T5–T10).
- Lesser splanchnic nerve (T10–T11).
- Least splanchnic nerve (T12).

What is the relation of the splanchnic nerves to the sympathetic trunk?

The splanchnic nerves are preganglionic sympathetic fibres that lie medial to the sympathetic trunk on the bodies of the thoracic vertebrae before traversing the diaphragm to innervate abdominal viscera.

What other longitudinal structure lies anterior to the thoracic sympathetic trunk on the left side of the thorax?

The thoracic duct.

19. Great Vessels

What are the branches of the arch of the aorta?
- Brachiocephalic trunk.
- Left common carotid artery.
- Left subclavian artery.

Do you know any variations in this pattern of branching?
Variation is so common that the normal pattern is only seen in approximately two-thirds of the population. In 5% of people, the left vertebral artery arises directly from the arch of the aorta, between the origins of the left common carotid and left subclavian arteries. More rare variations include: a left brachiocephalic artery which bifurcates to form the left common carotid and left subclavian arteries; a left common carotid arising from the brachiocephalic artery and an aberrant right subclavian artery arising distal to the left subclavian artery and passing to the right posteriorly to the oesophagus.

What are the branches of the descending aorta?
- Nine pairs of posterior intercostal arteries.
- One pair of subcostal arteries.
- Two to three bronchial arteries.
- Four to five oesophageal branches.
- Mediastinal branches.
- Phrenic branches.
- Pericardial branches.

What are the branches of the subclavian artery?
- Vertebral artery.
- Thyrocervical trunk.
- Internal thoracic artery.
- Costocervical trunk.
- Superior intercostal artery.

What are the branches of the thyrocervical trunk?
- Inferior thyroid artery.
- Transverse cervical artery.
- Suprascapular artery.

What are the tributaries of the brachiocephalic veins?
- Internal thoracic veins.
- Inferior thyroid veins.

On the left there is also the left superior intercostal vein and the thymic vein.

What are the landmarks of the cannulation of the subclavian vein?

The junction of the middle and medial thirds of the clavicle. The needle is placed below the clavicle aiming upwards and medially towards the sternoclavicular joint.

20. Oesophagus

Describe the peristaltic contractions seen in the oesophagus.

There are three types of peristaltic contractions seen in the oesophagus:

- Primary contractions which are initiated proximally by swallowing and progress distally pushing the bolus of food towards the stomach.
- Secondary contractions which are locally initiated waves along the length of the oesophagus clearing any matter left behind the food bolus.
- Tertiary contractions which are random, non-propulsive, uncoordinated contractions. Tertiary contractions increase with age and are the only form of peristalsis seen in achalasia.

What is the blood supply of the oesophagus?

The arterial supply is from the inferior thyroid artery, branches of the descending thoracic aorta and the left gastric artery. The cervical oesophagus drains into the inferior thyroid veins, the thoracic oesophagus drains into the azygous vein. The abdominal oesophagus drains via azygous and left gastric veins.

What is the lymphatic drainage of the oesophagus?

The lymphatic drainage is through the peri-oesophageal plexus to the posterior mediastinal nodes, which drain to the supraclavicular nodes and to the left gastric nodes.

What are the normal anterior indentations of the oesophagus seen on barium swallow?

The oesophagus is indented by the arch of the aorta, left bronchus and left atrium.

From what does the oesophagus develop?

The oesophagus develops from the primitive foregut which also forms the larynx and trachea.

Can you name some congenital abnormalities of the oesophagus?

- Oesophageal atresia.
- Tracheo-oesophageal fistula (1%).

21. Thoracic Duct

What is the course of the thoracic duct?

The thoracic duct arises from the cisterna chyli as it passes upwards through the right crus of the diaphragm immediately anterior to the vertebral bodies of L1 and L2. The thoracic duct then ascends behind the oesophagus in the right paravertebral space, crossing to the left at the level of T5. It runs alongside the upper oesophagus and behind the carotid sheath before descending over the left subclavian artery to drain into the start of the left brachiocephalic vein at the confluence of the left internal jugular and subclavian veins.

What anatomical territories does the thoracic duct drain?

Everything below the diaphragm and everything on the left hand side of the thorax and neck.

If the duct was damaged during an operation, e.g. block dissection of the neck, what should be done?

The injured duct should be ligated. Ideally, lymph will divert into the venous system via anastomoses. If this does not happen a chylous fistula neck may form in the neck.

Name four causes of chylothorax?

- Damage or obstruction of the thoracic duct.
- Carcinoma of the lung.
- Lymphoma.
- Tuberculosis.

If the thoracic duct was damaged in the upper part of the thorax what would be the likely side of a resulting chylothorax?

The left side. This is because as the thoracic duct passes up through the thorax it crosses from right to left at the level of T5. Disruption of the upper duct will produce a left chylothorax, while injury to the lower thoracic duct will produce a right chylothorax.

How do you confirm the diagnosis of a chylothorax?

The diagnosis is confirmed by triglyceride levels exceeding 110 mg/dl in the pleural fluid.

22. Diaphragm

How does the diaphragm develop?
The diaphragm develops in the cervical region of the embryo from four parts: the septum transversum, the pleuroperitoneal membranes, the body wall and the dorsal oesophageal mesentery. The septum transversum is carried ventrally and caudally so that in the adult it comes to lie in the anterior part of the diaphragm.

What is the innervation of the diaphragm?
Motor innervation is from the phrenic nerve (C3, C4 and C5). Sensory supply to the central portion of the diaphragm is also from the phrenic nerve. However, the periphery of the diaphragm receives its sensory supply from the lower six intercostal nerves.

What are the main openings in the diaphragm and what structures pass through them?
There are three main openings of the diaphragm:

1. The aortic opening, at the level of T12, which transmits the aorta, the thoracic duct and the azygous vein.
2. The oesophageal opening, at the level of T10, which transmits the oesophagus, the left gastric vessels and the vagus nerves.
3. The inferior vena caval opening, at the level of T8, which transmits the inferior vena cava and the right phrenic nerve.

What other structures pierce the diaphragm?
- Left phrenic nerve: pierces the central tendon.
- Splanchnic nerves (greater, lesser and least): pierce each crus.
- Sympathetic chain: passes behind the medial arcuate ligament.

How do you classify diaphragmatic hernias?
Diaphragmatic hernias may be congenital or acquired. There are four sites that congenital diaphragmatic hernia occur:

1. Through the foramen of Morgagni (located anteriorly between the xiphoid and costal origins).
2. Through the foramen of Bochdalek (a defect in the pleuroperitoneal canal).
3. Through a deficiency in the whole central tendon.
4. Through a congenitally large oesophageal hiatus.

Aquired diaphragmatic hernias may follow trauma the chest or abdomen. The left hemi-diaphragm is more affected than the right. Other acquired diaphragmatic hernias include sliding and rolling hiatal hernias.

ABDOMEN AND PELVIS

23. Anterior Abdominal Wall

What is the cutaneous nerve supply to the anterior abdominal wall?
- Seventh to twelfth intercostals nerves.
- The ileohypogastric nerve.

What is the lymphatic drainage of the anterior abdominal wall?
Above the umbilicus lymph drains upward to the axilla. Below the umbilicus lymph drains to the superficial inguinal nodes in the groin.

How can you divide the anterior abdominal wall into regions?
The anterior abdominal wall can be divided into regions by a grid of vertical and horizontal lines. The transpyloric plane lies horizontally on a line midway between the jugular notch and symphysis pubis. The transtuburcular plane also lies horizontally on a line through the tubercles of the iliac crests. The midclavicular planes provide a line on either side passing through the midclavicular point to midinguinal point.

How is the rectus sheath formed?
The rectus sheath encloses rectus abdominis and is formed by the aponeurotic tendons of the three lateral muscles: external oblique, internal oblique and transverses abdominis. The aponeurosis of these muscles joins together and then splits into the anterior and posterior layers of the rectus sheath around rectus abdominis. In the inferior part of the rectus sheath there is no posterior layer because all three aponeuroses pass anterior to rectus abdominis. The lower limit of the posterior layer of the rectus sheath is known as the arcuate line.

Can you describe the course of the inferior epigastric artery?
The inferior epigastric artery is a branch of the external iliac artery and passes upwards on the posterior abdominal wall medial to the deep inguinal ring. It then enters the rectus sheath at the arcuate line and then lies deep to rectus abdominis.

What forms the umbilical folds?
- Median umbilical fold: remnant of uracus.
- Medial umbilical folds: obliterated umbilical arteries.
- Lateral umbilical folds: inferior epigastric arteries.

24. Posterior Abdominal Wall

What structures make up the posterior abdominal wall?

Psoas major, quadratus lumborum, iliacus, the five lumbar vertebral bodies and their intervertebral discs.

What important ligaments lie on the posterior abdominal wall?

- Medial arcuate ligament: a thickening in psoas fascia between the L1 vertebra and the L1 transverse process.
- Lateral arcuate ligament: a thickening of fascia between the twelfth rib and the transverse process of L1.

What other structures lie immediately anterior to the posterior abdominal wall?

- Abdominal aorta.
- Inferior vena cava (IVC).
- Kidneys.
- Adrenal glands.
- Ureters.
- Sympathetic trunk.
- Subcostal nerve.
- Lumbar plexus.

What are the origins of the lumbar plexus?

L1–L4 ventral primary rami.

Which nerves arising from the lumbar plexus are associated anatomically with the posterior abdominal wall?

- Ileohypogastric nerve.
- Ileoinguinal nerve.
- Genitofemoral nerve.
- Lateral femoral cutaneous nerve of the thigh.
- Obturator nerve.
- Femoral nerve.

25. Inguinal Canal

Where does the inguinal ligament run?

From the anterior superior iliac spine to the pubic tubicle.

What are the boundaries of the inguinal canal?

The anterior wall is formed by the extensor oblique aponeurosis. The posterior wall is formed by the conjoint tendon and transversalis fascia. The roof is formed by the internal oblique and transversalis muscles. The floor is formed by the inguinal ligament and lacunar ligament.

What are the contents of the inguinal canal in males?

- The spermatic cord.
- Ileoinguinal nerve.

What is the surface marking of the deep inguinal ring?

The deep ring is just above the midpoint of the inguinal ligament.

What are the relations of the deep ring?

The deep ring is an opening in transversalis abdominis which borders the opening laterally and superiorly. Medially is transversalis fascia and the inferior epigastric artery.

Where is the superficial inguinal ring located?

It lies above and medial to the pubic tubicle. It is formed by a triangular gap in the fibres of external oblique.

26. Transpyloric Plane of Addison

At what level is the transpyloric plane?

It is at the lower level of L1.

What are the surface marking for the transpyloric plane?

It is midway between the jugular notch and symphysis pubis.

What structures are found in this plane?

- Fundus of the gall bladder.
- Pylorus of the stomach.
- Neck of the pancreas.
- Hila of the kidneys.
- Duodeno-jejunal flexure.
- Origin of the superior mesenteric artery from the aorta.
- Termination of the spinal cord.

What investigation is shown in Figure 1?

Computed tomography (CT) scan through the transpyloric plane of Addisson.

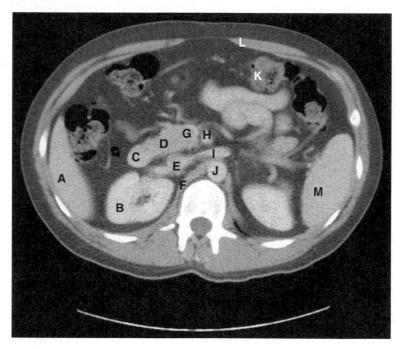

Figure 1.

Can you identify the structures A–M in Figure 1?

A Liver
B Right kidney
C Duodenum
D Pancreas
E IVC
F Right crus of the diaphragm
G Superior mesenteric vein

H Superior mesenteric artery
I Left renal vein
J Aorta
K Transverse colon
L Rectus abdominis
M Spleen

27. Stomach

Can you name the different parts of the stomach?

- Fundus.
- Cardia.
- Body.
- Pylorus.

What is attached to the lesser and greater curve of the stomach?
- Lesser curve: the lesser omentum.
- The greater curve: the greater omentum.

What are the anterior relations of the stomach?
The anterior abdominal wall, left costal margin and diaphragm.

What are the posterior relations of the stomach?
- The lesser sac.
- Diaphragm.
- Left suprarenal gland.
- Upper pole of left kidney.
- Pancreas.
- Left colic flexure.

What is the arterial supply to the stomach?
- Left gastric artery (from the coeliac trunk).
- Right gastric artery (from the hepatic artery).
- Left gastro-epiploic artery (from the splenic artery).
- Right gastro-epiploic artery (from gastro-duodenal artery).
- Short gastric artery (from the splenic artery).

28. Duodenum

Can you describe the course of the duodenum?
The duodenum forms a "C"-shape around the head of the pancreas from the pylorus of the stomach to the jejunum. The first part of the duodenum passes horizontally across the midline at the level of L1. It then descends vertically to the level of L3 before passing back horizontally across the midline to the left. The final part continues to the left ascending obliquely to the duodeno-jejunal flexure just below the level of L1.

Is the duodenum retroperitoneal?
Not completely: the first 2 cm is mobile and attached to the lesser omentum, the remainder is retroperitoneal.

What is the ligament of Treitz?
The ligament of Treitz is a band of connective tissue and smooth muscle passing from the right crus of the diaphragm to the duodeno-jejunal flexure which it supports.

What is the duodenal recesses?

There are several folds of peritoneum associated with the duodenum just before it reaches the duodeno-jejunal flexure. These folds form recesses: the paraduodenal recess, superior duodenal recess and the inferior duodenal recess.

Why is knowledge of these recesses important?

They are sites at which an internal hernia can occur.

29. Pancreas

Can you name the different parts of the pancreas?

- Head.
- Uncinate process.
- Body.
- Neck.
- Tail.

Where does the pancreas lie?

The pancreas lies at the level of the transpyloric plane (L1) running obliquely from the head, which lies in the "C"-shaped duodenum, to the tail behind the peritoneum on the posterior abdominal wall.

What are the posterior relations of the pancreas?

- Aorta.
- IVC.
- Right and left renal veins.
- Gastroduodenal artery.
- Commencement of portal vein.
- Splenic vein.
- Left crus of diaphragm.
- Left psoas.
- Left suprarenal gland.
- Hilum of left kidney.

What are the anterior relations of the pancreas?

- Transverse mesocolon.
- Stomach.
- Lesser sac.

What is the lienorenal ligament?

The lienorenal ligament is a fold of peritoneum containing the tail of the pancreas and the splenic vessels.

How does the pancreatic duct open into the duodenum?

There are two openings. The major pancreatic duct of Wursung opens through the ampulla of Vater. There is also an accessor pancreatic duct of Santorini which opens through the minor duodenal papilla more proximally in the duodenum.

30. Gall Bladder

What is the surface marking of the gall bladder?

The tip of the gall bladder is said to be located at the right costal margin in the midclavicular line. However, this contractile organ has a highly varied position.

What is the blood supply to the gall bladder?

The cystic artery which is a branch of the right hepatic is the principal supply however numerous small branches reach the organ from the liver bed.

What is a gallstone ileus and why does it occur?

Gallstone ileus is the passage of a gallstone into the small bowel that impacts in the terminal ileum (the narrowest part of the small bowel). This typically occurs after an episode or repeated attacks of cholecystitis. The gall bladder becomes adherent to either the duodenum or the transverse colon (its inferior relations) and a gallstone fistulates through into the gastrointestinal tract. If this occurs in the large bowel it rarely causes problems. However, in the small bowel it may cause an incomplete obstruction. An abdominal film may show the offending gallstone, reveal small bowel obstruction or air in the biliary tree.

What is Calot's triangle?

Calot's triangle is a triangle formed by the inferior surface of the liver, the cystic duct and the common hepatic duct. It is within the triangle than one can usually find the cystic artery. It is this piece of anatomy that surgeons seek to identify in performing cholecystectomy so that the cystic duct and artery can be safely tied off and cut without causing injury to the common bile duct.

What investigation is shown in Figure 2?

Endoscopic retrograde cholangiopancreatography (ERCP).

Can you identify structures A–E in Figure 2?

A   Gallstones in gall bladder

B   Duodenum

C   Cystic duct
D   Right hepatic duct
E   Left hepatic duct

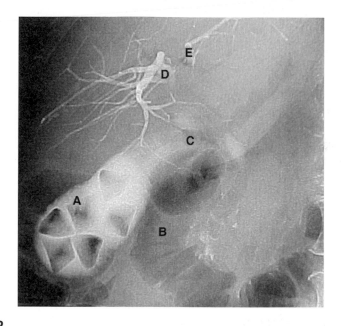

Figure 2.

What investigation is shown in Figure 3?

Percutaneous transhepatic cholangiogram (PTC).

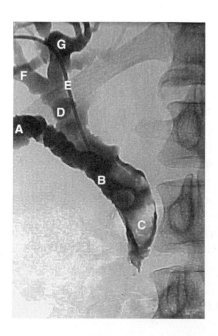

Figure 3.

Can you identify the structures labelled A–G in Figure 3?

A Cystic duct
B Common bile duct
C Impacted stones in common bile duct
D Common hepatic duct
E PTC catheter
F Right hepatic duct
G Left hepatic duct

31. Kidneys

What important layers surround the kidney substance?

The kidney tissue itself is enclosed within its own capsule. Outside this the perinephric fat encompasses both the kidney and its ipsilateral adrenal gland. Gerota's fascia then compartmentalises the adrenal and the kidney separately. The last immediate layer is composed of pararenal fat, which is more prominent posteriorly.

What are the important posterior relations of the kidney?

- Three important muscles: transversus abdominus, psoas major and quadratus lumborum.
- Three important nerves: subcostal nerve; ileohypogastric nerve; and ileoinguinal nerve.
- The diaphragm.

What are the important anterior relations of the left kidney?

- Stomach.
- Body of the pancreas.
- Spleen.
- Splenic flexure of the large bowel.
- Left adrenal.
- Descending colon.

What are the important anterior relations of the right kidney?

- Right lobe of the liver.
- Gall bladder.
- Hepatic flexure of the large bowel.
- Right adrenal.
- Second part of the duodenum.

What is the blood supply to the kidney?

Both the right and left renal arteries arise directly from the aorta. Several small veins come together to form the renal veins on each side which both drain directly into the IVC.

Why may a left-sided varicocoele be a presenting feature of a left-sided renal cell carcinoma?

Thrombosis of the left renal vein may be a complication of a left renal mass. Since the left gonadal vein drains into the left renal vein this thrombosis can result in varicosities of the pampiniform plexus. This clinical picture does not occur on the right because the right gonadal vein drains directly into the IVC.

What are the important structures entering and leaving the hila of the kidney and how are they related?

From anterior to posterior: the renal vein, the renal artery and the ureter.

From what important embryological structure is the kidney derived?

The kidney develops from a bud of tissue derived from the metanephric duct. The duct itself differentiates to form the ureter, renal pelvis and the collecting system of the kidney.

32. Intestines

What are the key differences between the jejunum and ileum?

The jejunum has thicker walls, thicker valvulae coniventes, a wider lumen, more villi, more plicae circlures and fewer arterial cascades than the ileum.

What are Peyer's patches?

Aggregations of lymphoid tissue in the lower ileum.

What features distinguish the large intestine from the small intestine?

1. Three flattened longitudinal muscle bands known as taeniae coli.
2. Appendices epiploicae.
3. Larger diameter lumen.

What is the arterial supply of the large bowel?

The superior and inferior mesenteric arteries.

Which parts of the large bowel do not have mesenteries?

The ascending and descending colon do not have true mesenteries in 90% of people. However, they form pseudomesenteries through the process of zygosis.

What is the surgical significance of knowing this?

The ascending and descending colon can usually be mobilised from the posterior abdominal wall swiftly with little risk of haemorrhage.

33. Aorta

At what level does the aorta enter the abdomen?

The aorta passes behind the diaphragm at the level of the twelfth thoracic vertebra (T12).

What structures accompany it at this level?

The azygous vein and thoracic duct.

At what level does the abdominal aorta terminate?

It bifurcates into common iliac arteries anterior to the body of the L4 vertebra.

What are the anterior relations of the abdominal aorta?

- Body of pancreas.
- Splenic vein.
- Left renal vein.
- Third part of duodenum.
- Loops of small bowel.

What is the diameter of the normal aorta?

The diameter of the normal aorta is 2 cm.

What are the main branches of the abdominal aorta?

- Visceral branches (paired): suprarenal, renal and gonadal.
- Anterior branches to the gut: coeliac, superior mesenteric and inferior mesenteric.
- Inferior phrenic arteries (paired).
- Lumbar arteries (paired).
- Terminal branches: left and right common iliac and median sacral artery.

34. Inferior Vena Cava

Can you tell me where the IVC originates?

The common iliac veins join at the level of the fifth lumbar vertebra behind the right common iliac artery to form the IVC.

At what level does the IVC pierce the diaphragm?

Level of the eighth thoracic vertebra (T8).

What are the surface markings of the IVC?

The IVC can be traced by a vertical line extending superiorly from 2.5 cm to the right of the midline at the level of intertubercular plane to the right sixth costal cartilage.

Does the liver drain directly into the IVC?

Yes. The IVC grooves the posterior surface of the liver where it receives three hepatic branches.

Can you tell me how the gonadal veins terminate?

The right gonadal vein drains directly into the IVC. The left drains into the left renal vein which then joins the IVC.

35. Scrotum and Testes

In performing scrotal surgery can you tell me the layers you would traverse before reaching the testis?

- Scrotal skin.
- Dartos muscle in superficial fascia.
- External spermatic fascia.
- Cremesteric muscle in cremesteric fascia.
- Internal spermatic fascia.
- Parietal layer of tunica vaginalis.
- Visceral layer of tunica vaginalis.
- Tunica albuginea of testis.

What is the appendix epididymis (hydatid of Morgagni)?

This is a small stalk-like structure found on the upper extremity of the epididymis. A similar structure, if found on the testis, is known as the appendix testis. They are both embryological remnants: the hydatid of Morgagni is a remnant of the mesonephros and the appendix testis is a remnant of the paramesonephric duct.

What is the significance of the appendix epididymis to testicular torsion?

In testicular torsion it is in fact the appendix of the epididymis that is usually the nidus for torsion.

What is the arterial supply to the testis?

The testes are supplied by the testicular arteries which arise on each side directly from the aorta. The artery of the vas, supplying the vas deferens and epididymis, is derived from the inferior vesicular branch from the internal iliac system. There is a rich anastomosis between the two.

What is the lymphatic drainage of the testis?

The testes drain to the para-aortic lymph nodes. The scrotum drains to the inguinal region.

What is the difference between a retractile testis and an undescended testis?

A retractile testis is a testis that does not lie within the scrotum but, on gentle manipulation, can be persuaded to return to its normal position. An undescended testis, on the other hand, is a testis that has failed to descend and has halted somewhere along the line of its descent.

36. Axilla

What do you understand by the term axilla?
The axilla is the space between the upper arm and the side of the thorax, anteriorly and posteriorly bounded by axillary folds. It communicates with the posterior triangle of the neck containing neurovascular structures and lymph nodes.

What are its anatomical boundaries?
Inferiorly the floor is comprised of axillary fascia running from serratus anterior to the deep fascia of the arm. The anterior wall contains pectoralis major, pectoralis minor, subclavius and the clavipectoral fascia. The posterior wall comprises subscapularis, teres major and the tendon of latissimus dorsi. The medial wall is formed by the upper part of serratus anterior. The lateral margin is formed by the medial border of the humerus.

What structures are contained within the axilla?
- Axillary artery.
- Axillary vein.
- Cords and terminal branches of the brachial plexus.
- Lymph nodes.
- Fat.

What is the surgical significance of pectoralis minor in breast surgery?
Pectoralis minor demarcates the three levels of axillary node clearance: level I is lateral to pectoralis minor; level II is up to the medial border of pectoralis minor and level III is medial to the medial border of pectoralis minor.

In operations involving the axilla what should be discussed when obtaining patient consent?
The patient should be warned of the possibility of neurovascular damage, e.g. damage to the axillary artery and brachial plexus. In particular, specific mention should be made of the risk of post-operative numbness on the medial aspect of the upper arm due to division of the intercostobrachial nerve. Other nerves that may be damaged include the long thoracic nerve to serratus anterior and the thoracodorsal nerve to latissimus dorsi.

37. Shoulder Joint

What type of joint is the shoulder joint?

A synovial ball and socket joint between the glenoid fossa of the scapula and the head of the humerus.

What are the characteristics of synovial joint of this type?

The joint cavity is filled with synovial fluid secreted from the synovial membrane inside the joint capsule. The joint surfaces are lined with hyaline cartilage. The joint itself is multi-axial with three planes of movement.

The shoulder joint is commonly dislocated where as the hip joint, a similar joint, dislocates relatively infrequently. Why is this?

The shoulder joint due is inherently less stable than the hip. The glenoid is less concave and the relative size of the head of the humerus compared to the glenoid is much greater than the ratio of the head of the femur to the acetabulum.

What provides stability to the shoulder joint?

The glenoid has a fibrocartilaginous labrum increasing the total articular surface area of the joint. Inside the capsule itself there are three gleno-humeral ligaments which strengthen the capsule. The most significant support comes from the intrinsic tone provided by the rotator cuff muscle: teres minor, infraspinatus, supraspinatus and subscapularis.

Clinically how would you diagnose shoulder dislocation?

Usually, the mechanism of injury will indicate the type of dislocation. The shoulder commonly dislocates anteriorly following a fall on a backwardly out-stretched hand. The shoulder contour is lost, or flattened, and a small bulge may be palpable just below the clavicle. A posterior dislocation results from forced internal rotation. The patient will hold the arm in internal rotation and will be unable to externally rotate the arm due to impingement of the humeral head on the glenoid.

What neurovascular structures are at risk in an anterior dislocation?

The axillary nerve as it winds around the surgical neck of the humerus. The axillary artery may also be damaged, therefore the limb should be examined for signs of ischaemia.

38. Brachial Plexus

What do you understand by the term plexus in relation to nerves?

A plexus is a network formed from anterior primary rami of spinal nerves dedicated to the supply of the skin and muscles of a vertebrates limb.

What are the root values of the brachial plexus?

The brachial plexus is formed from the anterior primary rami of C5, C6, C7, C8 and T1.

The anterior primary rami form the brachial plexus, what is the function of the posterior rami?

The posterior rami innervate the muscles of the back (known functionally as the erector spinae muscles) and supply sensation to the skin over the medial back.

How is the brachial plexus structurally arranged?

Anterior primary roots leave the intervertebral foraminae between scalenus anterior and scalenus medius to enter the base of the posterior triangle of the neck. The roots then form three trunks: upper (C5 and C6); middle (C7) and lower (C8 and T1). These trunks pass over the first rib posterior to third part of the subclavian artery. Each trunk then divides into an anterior and posterior division behind the clavicle. The divisions come together to form three cords named according to their relation to the axillary artery: lateral cord, medial cord and posterior cord. The cords then give rise to the five main nerves of the upper limb: axillary nerve, radial nerve, median nerve, ulnar nerve and musculocutaneous nerve.

The upper limb is a compartmentalised structure, how does its innervation reflect this?

Each compartment of the upper limb has a specific terminal branch of the brachial plexus supplying it. The posterior (extensor) compartments of the arm and forearm are supplied by the radial nerve (C5–T1). The flexor compartment of the arm is supplied by the musculocutaneous nerve (C5, C6 and C7), and the forearm flexor compartment is supplied (mainly) by the median nerve (C6, C7, C8 and T1). The ulnar nerve supplies the majority of the intrinsic muscles of the hand.

39. Blood Supply of Upper Limb

Through which structures does arterial blood reach the upper limb?

On the left side the subclavian artery takes origin directly from the aortic arch, while on the right it is a branch of the brachiocephalic trunk. The subclavian artery then becomes the axillary artery at the lateral border of the first rib, this then becomes the brachial artery at the lateral border of teres major. The brachial artery gives of a profunda brachii branch to supply structures in the upper arm. The brachial artery divides into two main terminal branches ulnar and radial arteries usually in the cubital fossa.

How is arterial blood supplied to the hand?

There are two palmar arches, a deep arch at the level of the base of the fully abducted thumb formed mainly from the radial artery. The superficial branch is formed from the termination of the ulnar artery and is at the level of the distal margin of the fully abducted thumb. There exist anastomoses between the two arches and hence between the two arteries.

Where would you take an arterial blood gas sample in the upper limb and what is the major risk associated with it?

Commonly from the radial artery at the wrist, although the ulnar artery may be used. As there is a risk of thrombosis of the vessel and hence distal ischaemia the brachial artery tends to be avoided as it represents the only main vessel supplying the arm.

Given this possible what tests would you perform to ensure that this would be safe?

Prior to taking a radial arterial sample I would perform Allen's test, to assess the adequacy of collateral circulation to the hand. By occluding both ulnar and radial arteries through digital pressure and the patient clenching the fist, on release of pressure over the artery palmar flushing should be seen within 15 seconds, indicating adequate collateral circulation.

What role may the upper limb vasculature play in the management of chronic lower limb ischaemia?

In patients with severe chronic lower limb ischaemia with pain present at rest where angioplasty has been unsuccessful or unviable surgical intervention is indicated necessitating a bypass. Patients with such symptoms often have co-morbid cardiac problems which may preclude major invasive bypass operations. In such cases extra-anatomical bypass procedures may be performed using the axillary artery: namely an axillo-bifemoral bypass.

40. Carpal Tunnel

What is the carpal tunnel?
An osteofascial compartment formed by the concavity of the carpal bones and bridged by the flexor retinaculum.

What are the attachments of the flexor retinaculum?
The tubercles on the scaphoid and trapezium on the radial side, and the pisiform and hamate on the ulnar side.

What are the contents of the carpal tunnel?
Ten tendons: four slips of flexor digitorum profundus, four slips of flexor digitorum superficialis, the tendon of flexor pollicis longus and the tendon of flexor carpi radialis.
   The median nerve lies in the midline superiorly.

What are the other neurovascular relationships to the carpal tunnel?
The radial and ulnar arteries run superficially over the carpal tunnel on their respective sides. The ulnar nerve which supplies most of the intrinsic muscles of the hand runs on the ulnar side of the ulnar artery superficially over the retinaculum to enter the hypothenar eminence.

What is carpal tunnel syndrome?
Carpal tunnel syndrome is characterised by a disturbance in median nerve function as it passes through the carpal tunnel. There are a variety of causes which result in compression of the median nerve as it passes through the carpal tunnel. Decompression of the carpal tunnel is, therefore, the rationale behind surgical management of carpal tunnel syndrome.

Is there any anatomical way of localising the problem to the carpal tunnel rather than more proximally in the median nerves course?
The lesion can be localised to the carpal tunnel if skin sensation over the thenar eminence is preserved. Sensation in this area is supplied by the palmar cutaneous branch, which, originating from the median nerve proximal to the flexor retinaculum, does not pass through the carpal tunnel and hence avoids compression.

What other median nerve neuropathies in the arm are you aware of?

- Pronator syndrome: due to median nerve compression at the elbow by structures such as the ligament of struthers, the proximal arch of flexor digitorum superficialis, or pronator teres.
- Anterior interosseous syndrome: entrapment of the nerve by the deep head of pronator teres causes weakness in the radial half of flexor digitorum profundus, flexor pollicis longus and pronator quadratus.

41. Femoral Triangle

What are the boundaries of the femoral triangle?

- Superiorly: inguinal ligament and body of pubis.
- Laterally: medial border sartorius.
- Medially: medial border adductor longus.
- Floor: iliacus, tendon of psoas, pectineus and adductor longus.
- Roof: fascia lata.

What anatomical structures are found in the femoral triangle?

- Femoral vein, artery and nerve (from medial to lateral in the femoral sheath).
- Great saphenous vein entering the femoral vein.
- Deep inguinal lymph nodes.

What pathological structures may be found in the femoral triangle?

- Femoral hernia.
- Saphena varix.
- Enlarged lymph nodes.
- Femoral aneurysm.

How would you locate and palpate the femoral artery?

The femoral artery is found at the midinguinal point, i.e. midway between the anterior superior iliac spine and the pubic symphysis. The artery is palpated by compression against the superior pubic ramus.

What is the relationship of the deep inguinal ring to the femoral artery?

The deep ring lies just lateral to the deep ring at the midpoint of the inguinal ligament. Midway between the anterior superior iliac spine and the ipsilateral pubic tubercle.

How would you locate the saphenous opening in a high-saphenous ligation (Trendelenberg operation)?

Three centimetres below and lateral to the pubic tubercle, usually access achieved by a transverse skin incision.

42. Popliteal Fossa

What are the margins of the popliteal fossa?

The popliteal fossa is a diamond-shaped space on the posterior aspect of the knee. The upper margins are comprised laterally by biceps femoris tendon and medially by semimembranosus with semitendinosus. The lower borders are the medial and lateral heads of gastrocnemius. The roof is formed of the fascia lata.

What structures are found in the popliteal fossa?

The artery is the deepest structure with the popliteal vein overlying it. The tibial nerve lies superficial to the vein. The common peroneal nerve lies in the lateral aspect of the fossa following the medial edge of the biceps tendon. The remaining space is filled with fat and popliteal lymph nodes.

What is the origin of the popliteal artery?

The femoral artery passes through the adductor or Hunter's canal between the adductor and hamstring parts of the adductor magnus muscle into the popliteal fossa. At this point the femoral artery becomes the popliteal artery.

What is the surgical significance of the popliteal fossa in terms of the venous drainage?

The short saphenous vein perforates the roof of the fossa through the deep fascia to enter the popliteal vein, representing a major point of drainage of the superficial venous system into the deep system. It is the location for short saphenous ligation and stripping when varicosities are present.

What pathological lumps may be commonly felt in the fossa?

- Popliteal aneurysm.
- Baker's cyst.
- Varicosities of the short saphenous vein.
- Lymph nodes.
- Lipoma.
- Sarcoma.
- Tend.
- Tendinous bursae.

43. Hip Joint

What sort of joint is the hip joint?
A synovial ball and socket joint.

What structures comprise the hip joint?
- The head of the femur.
- The acetabulum (formed from the confluence of the ischial, pubic and iliac bones).
- A joint capsule.
- The acetabular labrum (a fibrocartilaginous rim strengthened inferiorly by the transverse ligament).
- The Haversian fat pad.
- Three ligaments originating from each constituent of the acetabulum spiralling down the long axis of the neck of the femur: pubofemoral ligament, ileofemoral ligament and the ischiofemoral ligament.
- Ligamentum teres.

Where does the capsule of the hip joint adhere to the femoral neck?
Anteriorly the capsule extends from the intertrochanteric line to the acetabular rim. Posteriorly the capsule extends from half-way up the femoral neck to the acetabular rim.

The shoulder and hip joint are of the same type both with large degrees of movement. However the shoulder joint may easily dislocate where as the hip does so infrequently. How is this balance of stability and mobility achieved anatomically?
Broadly speaking, stability comes from the adaptation of the articular surfaces: the acetabulum and labrum enclose the head of the femur securely. Freedom results from the neck of the femur being much narrower than the maximal diameter of the head.

How is blood supplied to the head of the femur and does it change throughout life?
The main supply is through the trochanteric anastomoses. The lateral and medial circumflex femoral arteries send branches which pass along the neck of the femur beneath the retinacular fibres of the capsule. In the adult there may also be supply through the neck itself from the shaft of the femur once the epiphysis has closed. In the infant and child supply through the artery in the ligamentum teres (a branch of the obturator) is significant.

What is the surgical significance of the blood supply to the head of the femur?

Fractures that are intracapsular in the adult will result in devascularisation of the head of the femur. The end result of this is avascular necrosis.

44. Compartments of the Leg

How are the muscles of the leg grouped anatomically?

They are compartmentalised with muscles of a similar action and are grouped into osseofascial compartments.

What specific structures provide this arrangement?

The whole limb is enclosed in a sleeve of deep fascia known as the fascia lata. Intermuscular septa run from the deep surface of the fascia lata to attach to the lower limb bones, thereby dividing the limb into muscular compartments.

How does this organisation relate to neurovascular structures in the leg?

Each compartment has it own specific artery and nerve to supply the musculature.

What problem can the enclosure in these osteofascial compartments cause after trauma?

Compartment syndrome: due to compression of the enclosed structures due to swelling within the enclosed compartment.

How is this condition managed?

By fasciotomy to decompress the fascial compartment.

45. Innervation of Lower Limb

What are the three major nerves supplying lower limb structures?

The femoral nerve (L2, L3 and L4), the obturator nerve (L2, L3 and L4), and the sciatic nerve (L4, L5, S1, S2 and S3), all originating from the lumbosacral plexus.

How do the anterior primary rami of these nerves reach the lower limb structures which they innervate?

The femoral and obturator nerves form from the anterior and posterior divisions of the anterior first-degree rami around the psoas muscle. The femoral nerve emerges laterally and passes across the iliac fossa to enter the thigh beneath the inguinal ligament lateral to the femoral artery. The obturator nerve emerges from the medial aspect of psoas and passes behind the iliac vessels to exit via the obturator foramen. The sciatic nerve is formed from the lumbosacral trunk running over psoas that joins S1, S2 and S3 to lie on the surface of piriformis. From here it passes through the greater sciatic foramen to enter the leg.

Can you explain the role of the sciatic nerve in a Trendelenberg gait?

The sciatic nerve gives off the superior gluteal nerve in the buttock area to supply gluteus medius and minimis. Damage to this nerve results in failure of the abductor mechanism of the hip. The result of this is that, during the swing phase of walking on the affected side, the contralateral pelvis falls below horizontal as the ipsilateral gluteal muscles fail to adduct the ipsilateral ischial crest.

Are there any other conditions where a high-stepping gait is indicative of damage to another terminal branch of the sciatic nerve?

The sciatic nerve divides at a variable point in the hamstring compartment into the tibial and common peroneal nerves. The common peroneal nerve innervates the dorsiflexors and everters of the foot. Damage to the common peroneal nerve, e.g. from direct trauma in the popliteal fossa, can result in a foot drop. This may present as a high-stepping gait to avoid dragging the toes on the floor.

How is the sciatic nerve commonly damaged in the upper thigh, how does this affect clinical practice?

Iatrogenic injuries through intramuscular (IM) injections represent the commonest form of damage. The nerve exits in the lower medial quadrant and IM injections are given in the upper outer quadrant to avoid this.

What part of the lower limb receives its sensory supply from the deep peroneal nerve?

The first dorsal web space of the foot between the great and second toe.

What part of the lower limb receives its sensory supply from the superficial peroneal nerve?

The dorsum of the foot except for the first dorsal web space.

What is the dermatomal root value for sensation on the lateral side of the foot?

The dermatomal root value is S1.

What part of the lower limb receives its sensory supply from the saphenous nerve?

The medial side of the lower leg (the gaiter area).

What muscles are supplied by the deep peroneal nerve?

- Tibialis anterior.
- Extensor digitorum longus.
- Extensor hallucis longus.

What muscles are supplied by the superficial peroneal nerve?

Peroneus longus and brevis.

HEAD AND NECK

THORAX AND BREAST

ABDOMEN AND PELVIS

LUMPS AND BUMPS

LIMBS

1. Salivary Glands

What important structures lie within the parotid gland?

- Facial nerve.
- Retro-mandibular vein.
- External carotid artery – bifurcating into its two terminal branches, the maxillary artery and the superficial temporal artery.

Can you outline the surface markings of the parotid gland for?

Using a marker begin a line from in front of the tragus of the ear and draw it into the middle of the cheek below the zygomatic arch. From here proceed downwards and backwards to a point 1 cm in front of the angle of the mandible. Then continue upwards and backwards 1–2 cm into the neck including the mastoid process. Finally draw your line around the ear to join up to the point from where we started. You will now have drawn a shape that approximates the position of the parotid.

What are the potential complications of parotid surgery?

- Facial nerve damage.
- Haematoma.
- Frey's syndrome (gustatory sweating).
- Numbness of the pinna (due to sacrifice of the greater auricular nerve).
- Salivary fistula (in superficial parotidectomy only, as the cut gland left behind continues to secrete saliva).
- Wound dimple.

During surgery how would you locate the facial nerve?

This can be done in three different ways:

1. by identifying the tip of the tragal cartilage with during the dissection – the facial nerve lies 1 cm inferior and deep to this cartilage;
2. by locating the posterior belly of digastric and tracing this backwards to the tympanic plate – the facial nerve can be found between these two structures;
3. by locating the posterior facial vein at the inferior aspect of the gland – the marginal branch of the facial nerve will be seen crossing it.

Can you explain Frey's syndrome?

Frey's syndrome is excessive sweating, facial flushing, with or without pain, in the distribution of the auriculotemporal nerve. It is caused by sympathetic secreto-motor fibres arising from the auriculotemporal nerve, severed during surgery, reinnervating the facial skin (mainly the anterior skin flap formed by the incision).

What nerves are at risk while performing submandibular gland surgery?

- Mandibular branch of the facial nerve.
- Hypoglossal nerve.
- Lingual nerve.

How does one minimise the risk of damage to the marginal mandibular branch of the facial nerve?

The incision in submandibular surgery is made parallel and inferior to the mandible at the level of the hyoid bone or 2–3 fingerbreadths below the mandible. This will ensure safe approach to the gland with minimum risk of damage to the nerve.

What would be the effect of severing the lingual and hypoglossal nerves in surgery?

Lingual nerve damage results in ipsilateral loss of somatic sensation and taste to the anterior two-thirds of the tongue. Hypoglossal nerve damage results in ipsilateral paralysis and wasting of the muscles of the tongue. The tongue will deviate to the side of lesion when it is protruded.

2. Thyroidectomy

When consenting patients for thyroidectomy, what important risks should the patient be informed of?

Patients should be informed of the risks of: infection, haemorrhage with the potential for airway compromise, recurrent laryngeal nerve damage, external laryngeal nerve damage, hypothyroidism and hypocalcaemia secondary to parathyroid bruising or removal.

Describe how you would make the incision for a total thyroidectomy?

The incision should be approximately two fingerbreadths above the

suprasternal notch.

What layers will be breached in your approach to the thyroid gland?

- Skin.
- Subcutaneous fat.
- Platysma in the investing layer of fascia.
- Strap muscles (sternohyoid and sternothyroid).
- Pretracheal fascia.
- Isthmus of the thyroid gland.

What vessels need to be ligated to prevent bleeding and aid delivery of the gland?

The superior and inferior thyroid arteries and the superior, middle and inferior thyroid veins. It is advisable to secure the upper pole first as this will facilitate delivery of the gland into the surgical field.

What important nerve bears a close relation to the superior pole?

The external laryngeal nerve. Inadvertent damage to this nerve will result in a hoarse voice.

How would you go about identifying the recurrent laryngeal nerve?

By identifying the inferior thyroid artery and following its path towards the inferior pole of the gland. As the artery arches forward the nerve should come into view. It is wise to remember that the nerve may pass below, above or through the branches of the artery.

What are the landmarks for identifying the parathyroid glands?

The superior parathyroid glands usually lie just below the middle of the gland where the recurrent laryngeal nerve crosses the inferior thyroid artery. The inferior glands are usually placed close to the inferior pole. Unfortunately, the position of the parathyroids is quite varied. It is particularly crucial to make sure they are visualised in a total thyroidectomy so as to avoid potentially life-threatening post-operative hypocalcaemia.

What is Berry's ligament?

The ligament of Berry is one of the last structures divided in total thyroidectomy. It is a strong ligament that attaches the posterior aspect of the thyroid gland to the trachea.

You are called to the recovery room 45 minutes after a total thyroidectomy. The patient is struggling to breathe and the oxygen saturations are dropping rapidly. What is the likely problem and how would you proceed?

The problem is likely to be haemorrhage with airway compromise from expanding haematoma. The dressings should be removed and the area assessed for swelling. If a haematoma is confirmed the clips/sutures will need removing immediately. Once the haematoma is decompressed the patient can be taken back to theatre for formal reexploration of the wound.

3. Burr-holes

Are burr-holes always indicated for chronic subdural haematoma?

No, in some cases chronic subdural haematomas may respond to a short course of steroids.

How many burr-holes are needed to drain a chronic subdural haematoma?

The number of burr-holes will depend on the size and location of the haematoma. For example, for a unilateral haematoma one burr-hole may suffice but two burr-holes allows saline to be washed through the subdural space to help evacuate the clot.

Are there any principles that should be adhered to when deciding upon the location of a burr-hole?

Burr-holes should be located away from the dural sinuses (e.g. >2.5 cm from midline to avoid sagittal sinus). If being placed for the drainage of a chronic subdural haematoma they should be located along the line of a trauma flap so that, if necessary, it is possible to proceed to craniotomy. It is also necessary to avoid placing burr-holes over eloquent cortical areas such as the motor strip.

What is the surface marking of the motor strip?

The motor strip is located about 4–5 cm posterior to the coronal suture. The motor strip can also be estimated by taking a point 2 cm posterior to the midpoint over the top of the skull in the midline between the nasion and inion.

For the insertion of an extraventricular cerebrospinal fluid (CSF) drain a burr-hole is made at Kocher's point: how is this point identified?

Kocher's point is located 1 cm anterior to the coronal suture in the midpupillary line (this is approximately 2.5 cm parallel to the midline). The coronal suture can be palpated through the scalp.

Describe briefly how you would make a burr-hole to drain a chronic subdural haematoma.

The patient is positioned supine on the operating table. The patient is shaved, prepared and draped at the site of the burr-hole. Local anaesthetic with adrenaline is infiltrated down to the periosteum. A 2–3-cm incision is made in the line of craniotomy flap over the site of the burr-hole. The periosteum is striped away from the bone. A self-retainer is inserted to hold the edges of the scalp back fine haemostasis of the scalp is achieved with the diathermy. The drill is used to cut through the bone by applying firm pressure but without leaning the body-weight on to it. Once the dura is exposed the blue of the subdural haematoma will be seen. Bleeding to bone can be controlled with bone wax. The dura is scorched with the diathermy and then incised using a blunt hook to lift it and the tip of a sharp knife to make a cruciate incision. The four leaves of the dura thus formed can then be shrunk back with the diathermy. If the membranes of the chronic subdural have not burst by this stage then they can be scorched with the diathermy and opened with a blunt instrument such as MacDonald.

4. Tracheostomy

Can you give three indications for a tracheostomy?
- Long-term mechanical ventilation (this is the commonest reason).
- To bypass airway obstruction caused by a congenital anomaly.
- Bilateral vocal cord paralysis.

How would you perform an open tracheostomy?

A 2–3-cm transverse incision is made 2 cm above the sternal notch. The deep fascia is divided and the infrahyoid muscles are separated. The thyroid isthmus is carefully exposed and adequate haemostasis achieved. The pretracheal fascia is divided to expose trachea down to the fourth tracheal ring. Before the trachea is incised a moment is taken to recheck that a correct sized tube is available.

The trachea is incised between either the second and third, or the third and fourth, tracheal rings.

Which anatomical structure is particularly at risk when performing a tracheostomy on a child?

The innominate vein because it lies high on the trachea in children.

What measures are taken post-operatively to manage the tracheostomy?

Humidified oxygen should be used and the tube should be irrigated with saline every 15 minutes to begin with. The use of mucolytic agents is sometimes required and the tube should be left in place for 5–7 days and then replaced.

What are the potential complications of a tracheostomy?

Immediate
- Apnoea: due to lowered hypoxic drive.
- Haemorrhage.
- Pneumothorax.

Early
- Tracheitis.
- Mucous plugging.
- Cellulitis.
- Displacement.
- Subcutaneous emphysema.

Late
- Bleeding: may be secondary to tracheo-innominate fistula if occurs >48 hours after the procedure.
- Tracheomalacia.
- Strictures.

5. Central Venous Access

What are the two main sites used for central venous access?

The internal jugular vein (IJV) and femoral vein are the two preferred sites. The use of the subclavian vein is not advised as the incidence of thrombosis approaches 50% and access is more difficult. When using the IJV the right side is preferred because of its straight course to the superior vena cava (SVC).

Describe the technique for accessing the IJV.

The percutaneous approach is the commonest. The patient should be positioned in the Trendelenberg position to minimise the risk of air embolus. The needle is inserted at 45 degrees to the skin surface and introduced lateral to the carotid artery pulsation between the two heads of the sternocleidomastoid muscle. The tip of the introducer is aimed towards the ipsilateral nipple. Once blood is drawn into the needle a guidewire is inserted down the lumen of the needle and a sheath is advanced over the surface of the guidewire. If there is any doubt as to the position of the IJV, or the vein has been used many times before, it is preferable to use an ultrasound-guided technique.

Why do patients require central venous access?

- For the administration of antibiotics and chemotherapeutic agents that would otherwise damage peripheral veins.
- Total parenteral nutrition.
- Haemodialysis.
- Plasmapheresis.
- Frequent blood sampling.
- Measurement of central venous pressure.
- To pass a Swan–Ganz catheter.

What are the complications of central venous access?

Early
- Arterial puncture.
- Pneumothorax/haemopneumothorax.
- Rupture of vein cannulated.
- Air embolus.
- Malpositioning of the catheter.
- Migration of the catheter.

- Cardiac dysrhythmia.
- Right ventricular infarction.

Late
- Catheter infection.
- Catheter occlusion, e.g. secondary to formation of thrombus.
- Catheter migration.
- Arteriovenous fistula.

6. Thoracotomy

What are the indications for an emergency thoracotomy?

Any penetrating thoracic injury causing a cardiac arrest with electrical activity present and unresponsive hypotension (defined as BP <70 mmHg), or blunt thoracic injury with unresponsive hypotension and rapid exsanguination through a chest tube >1500 ml.

Can you think of any situation where an emergency thoracotomy might not be reasonable in thoracic trauma?

Blunt thoracic injuries that are pulseless but still have myocardial electrical activity are not suitable. The majority of blunt thoracic injuries can be managed without the need for thoracotomy.

What are the therapeutic aims of a thoracotomy?
- Direct access to control massive intrathoracic haemorrhage.
- Release of cardiac tamponade.
- Open cardiac massage.
- Access to cross-clamp the descending aorta.

Describe the surgical approach for emergency thoracotomy.

In a supine patient, a left-sided anterolateral thoracotomy is performed through a skin incision in the fifth intercostal space extending from the sternal border to the midaxillary line. This incision is extended through subcutaneous tissue down to the intercostal muscles. The intercostal muscles taking care to ensure that lung tissue is not damaged. Rib spreaders are used to widen the opening into the chest. If access to the right side of chest is required then the same procedure can be repeated on the opposite side and the sternum divided with a saw.

7. Pleurocentesis

What are the clinical features of a pleural effusion?

Reduced chest expansion; stony dullness to percussion; reduced or absent breath sounds; reduced vocal resonance over the effusion; aegophony at the top of the effusion and mediastinal shift with large effusions.

What are the radiological features of a pleural effusion?

To detect an effusion radiologically there has to be at least 200–300 ml of fluid. On a plain chest X-ray there may only be blunting of the costophrenic angle. A small effusion can be differentiated from pleural thickening by using a lateral decubitus film, which will allow any fluid to collect as a puddle in the most dependant part of the thorax. Larger effusions have a concave upper border and a massive effusion may show mediastinal shift.

What are the possible causes of a pleural effusion?

The causes are usually divided into transudates or exudates depending on the protein content of any fluid removed. Transudates have protein levels <30 g/l and exudates have levels >30 g/l. Transudates may occur with disorders such as congestive cardiac failure, hepatic cirrhosis and nephrotic syndrome. Exudates may occur with disorders such as malignancy (mesothelioma, primary lung cancer and metastases), infections or intestinal disease (intra-abdominal abscess and pancreatitis).

Describe the technique for performing pleurocentesis of a pleural effusion.

The upper border of the effusion is percussed and an entry point chosen one or two intercostal spaces below this in the posterior axillary line. One percent of lignocaine (5–10 ml) is infiltrated down to the pleura. A 21-gauge needle is inserted just above the upper border of the rib. Twenty to thirty millilitres of fluid is aspirated to be sent for biochemistry, bacteriology, cytology and immunology if required. If the effusion is symptomatic then more fluid may be removed. Fluid is best removed slowly at a rate of 1–2 l/24 hours. This can be done by hand or by inserting a drain.

What are the potential complications of pleurocentesis?

- Pneumothorax.
- Subcutaneous haematoma.
- Infection of the pleural space.
- Splenic/hepatic laceration.

8. Mastectomy and Wide Local Excision

What is the blood supply to the breast?
- The axillary artery via its lateral thoracic and acromio-thoracic branches.
- The internal thoracic artery via its four perforator branches.
- Branches of the anterior intercostal arteries.

Where do the lymphatics of the breast drain to?
- Axillary nodes.
- Internal mammary nodes.
- Contralateral breast.
- Abdominal wall.

Generally speaking, lymphatics from the medial side of the breast spread to the internal mammary nodes, and those of the upper and lateral aspect of the breast drain to the axillary nodes.

What are the indications for performing breast conservation surgery over mastectomy for carcinoma?
- Small single tumours in a large breast.
- Peripheral location.
- Local disease with no extensive nodal involvement.

What are the operative principles of wide local excision?
Wide local excision encompasses lumpectomy, segmentectomy and quadrantectomy. Of these, quadrantectomy is the procedure of choice as it provides the widest clearance. The lump and the quadrant are marked out with a marker pen. The quadrant is marked such that the lump is centred between its edges. The quadrant edges begin at the nipple and extend towards the periphery with both lines being at right angles to each other. All macroscopic tumour is excised and at least a 2-cm margin of normal breast tissue surrounding is removed with the tumour. The specimen is orientated for the pathologist by marking the planes of the specimen are marked with suture material. The aim of the surgery is to ensure histological margins are clear of microscopic disease. Meticulous haemostasis is achieved and the cavity packed while proceeding to axillary dissection.

What layers will you traverse in your dissection of the tumour?
- Skin.
- Superficial fascia (modified fat of the breast).

- Upward continuation of Scarpa's fascia (above costal margin).
- Posterior capsule of the breast.
- Retro-mammary space.

What is the long-term survival difference between breast conservation surgery and mastectomy in treating breast carcinoma?

Five- to ten-year survival data indicate no difference in patients undergoing mastectomy or breast conservation such as quadrantectomy, axillary dissection plus radiotherapy. Local recurrence rates in the latter group are slightly higher but this group of patients have superior cosmetic results.

What are the important pathological prognostic factors in breast cancer?

- Tumour grade.
- Positive regional nodes.
- Multi-centric tumour within the breast.
- Vascular invasion.

9. Axillary Clearance

What are the important contents of the axilla?
- Fat.
- Lymph nodes.
- Axillary artery and vein.
- Cords of the brachial plexus.
- Nerve to serratus anterior.
- Long thoracic nerve.
- Intercostobrachial nerve.

In performing an axillary clearance what would be the consequence of sacrificing the intercostobrachial nerve?

Patients will develop an area of numbness in the axilla and upper medial aspect of their arm. This possibility should always be discussed with the patient.

What are the anatomical boundaries of the axilla?
- Apex: bounded by the outer border of the first rib medially, the middle third of the clavicle antero-laterally and by the upper border of the scapula posteriorly.

- Inferiorly: the fascial floor which runs between the anterior and posterior axillary folds. The floor is supported by the suspensory axillary ligament which gives the axilla its classical tented appearance.
- Medially: the chest wall.
- Laterally: intertubercular sulcus of the humerus and the biceps tendon.
- Anteriorly: pectoralis major and minor muscles.
- Posteriorly: subscapularis, teres major; latissimus dorsi and scapula.

What are the purposes of axillary clearance in breast tumour surgery?

- Staging of the tumour.
- For prognostic purposes.
- Removal of disease.

How are axillary nodes classified anatomically?

The axillary nodes are split into three levels: level I – lateral to pectoralis minor, level II – at the level or posterior to pectoralis minor and level III – medial to pectoralis minor.

To what level is axillary clearance usually performed?

A level II clearance provides satisfactory disease control in the vast majority of cases.

What is axillary node sampling?

Axillary node sampling involves removing a sample of nodes lateral to pectoralis minor muscle. This stages the axilla but patients require post-operative radiotherapy to the axilla as a formal clearance has not been performed. There is less morbidity when compared to axillary clearance but problems with sampling include understaging, lack of regional control and a higher recurrence rate.

What is a sentinel lymph node biopsy?

Sentinel lymph node biopsy involves the accurate localisation of the first axillary lymph node draining breast tissue involved with tumour. This involves radioisotopes and dye to accurately localise the sentinel node. Once this has been carried out the node is dissected out and examined. If this node is negative it makes it extremely unlikely for any other axillary lymph nodes to be positive. Sentinel lymph node biopsy reduces complications associated with axillary clearance and radiotherapy, namely nerve damage (nerve to serratus anterior, long thoracic nerve and intercostobrachial nerve), axillary vein damage and lymphoedema.

10. Abdominal Incisions

In performing a midline incision to open the abdomen what layers will you come across in your approach?

- Skin.
- Subcutaneous fat.
- Camper's fascia (lower abdomen).
- Scarpa's fascia.
- Linea alba.
- Fascia transversalis.
- Extraperitoneal fat.
- Parietal peritoneum.
- Abdominal cavity.

When the abdominal cavity is open, what can you see in the operative field?

- Stomach.
- Greater omentum with an impression of the small bowel loops underneath.
- Left lobe of the liver.

Sigmoid colon and small bowel loops may be in sight if the greater omentum has been removed by previous surgery.

What is the difference between a paramedian and a rectus-splitting incision?

A paramedian incision is a vertical incision approximately 2 cm lateral to the midline. The rectus muscle is dissected and the anterior sheath retracted laterally. The posterior sheath is incised along with the peritoneum to gain access to the abdominal cavity. In the rectus-splitting incision, as the name implies, the rectus muscle is cut to gain access. The medial fibres of the sheath lose their innervation and thus this part of the muscle atrophies. The rectus-splitting incision, once used in the upper right abdomen for gall bladder surgery, has now been superseded by the more common use of Kocher's incision or transverse for open cholecystectomy.

What incision would you use in performing an appendectomy?

A Lanz or gridiron incisions are commonly used. The Lanz incision is a transverse incision in the right iliac fossa. It commences approximately

2 cm below and medial to the anterior superior iliac spine. It has a cosmetic advantage as the incision is in a skin crease although inferior access is more difficult to establish. The gridiron incision is made at right angles to McBurney's point, a line one third of the way up from the anterior superior iliac spine towards the umbilicus.

How you would use "mass closure" to close the abdomen?

Mass closure is often employed to close a midline incision of the abdomen. The linea alba is closed in one layer, i.e. the peritoneum and rectus sheath are closed as one. Most common loop (polydioxanone) PDS is used with a curved-blunted needle at either end. One suture is secured at one end of the wound to encompass the peritoneum and rectus sheath. The needle is fed through the loop to secure the knot down. The preferred method is to grab the sheath with the forceps and place the suture through the sheath. Care is taken to ensure bowel is not caught in the first knot. Further bites are taken 1 cm from the edge of the sheath and 1 cm further up from the last knot. Each knot should be loose at this point. Again, at each level care is taken to ensure bowel is not being caught in the suture. When half-way down the wound suturing stops and the sutures tightened. The process is then repeated from the other end of the wound. When the two sutures meet in the middle, the needles are cut off both sutures. A finger sweep is performed to check one last time that there is no bowel caught in the suture. The two ends are then tied together. The skin is closed with either clips or a subcuticular suture of choice. The length of suture used for mass closure should be four times the length of the wound (Jenkins Rule).

11. Inguinal Hernia Repair

What the possible causes of a lump in the groin?
- Inguinal hernia.
- Femoral hernia.
- Saphena varix.
- Lipoma of the cord.
- Hydrocoele of the cord.
- Ectopic testes.
- Inguinal lymphadenopathy.
- Psoas abscess.
- Ileo-femoral aneurysm.
- Malgaigne's bulges.

How can you distinguish between a direct and an indirect inguinal hernia?

This can be done by clinical examination but not reliably. The only way to be sure, is at time of surgery. If the sac of the hernia emerges lateral to the inferior epigastric vessels, it is an indirect inguinal hernia. If the hernia is medial to the vessels it is a direct inguinal hernia.

How would you perform an open inguinal hernia repair using mesh?

Most open inguinal repairs are performed using the Lichtenstein technique. This is a tension-free technique which involves placement of a mesh to reinforce the posterior wall. An oblique incision is made parallel to, and 2 cm above, the inguinal ligament. The fascia is dissected to expose the external oblique aponeurosis. A small incision is made in the external oblique in the lines of its fibres. A finger is inserted into the plane underneath external oblique to locate the external ring. Using scissors, the external oblique aponeurosis is cut in the line of its fibres towards the external ring until this is laid open. The opening in external obliques is now continued the other way in a similar fashion. An artery forceps is applied to each leaf of the cut external oblique. The spermatic cord is mobilised to develop a plane medially close to the pubic tubercle. The cord is encompassed with a cord clamp to isolate it. The cord is then displaced laterally with the use of some gauze or a cord clamp. A direct hernia will now become more obvious and, if apparent, can be dissected free and isolated. An indirect sac must be isolated from the cord. Firstly, the first layer of the cord is opened and each layer gently peeled with a combination of blunt and sharp dissection. A white curved edge will eventually be found which will represent the sac of the hernia. The sac is dissected free and picked up between two artery forceps. The sac can now be opened and any contents returned to the peritoneal cavity. The neck of the sac is transfixed and tied with synthetic absorbable suture, such as vicryl 2/0, but leave the suture ends uncut. Excise the sac before cutting the ligature. The stump of the sac should now be returned to the abdominal cavity.

A mesh repair is now performed by preshaping the mesh: the upper medial corner is cut to leave a curved border and a split is made in the mesh to facilitate the spermatic cord. Using a nylon suture, or non-absorbable equivalent, the mesh is secured ensuring good medial cover (the commonest site of recurrence). A medial suture is placed first and then the lateral border of the mesh is aligned with the inguinal ligament and sutured with a continuous suture. When the internal ring is approached the needle is passed underneath the cord. The suturing continued laterally, and then a knot secured. The medial and upper borders of the mesh are secured with interrupted sutures. The wound is closed in layers: external oblique using an absorbable suture such as vicryl, and then close the skin with a subcuticular vicryl suture. Local anaesthetic may be injected into the wound to help post-operative analgesia.

What are the National Institute for Clinical Excellence (NICE) guidelines for recurrent and bilateral inguinal hernias?

Bilateral and recurrent inguinal hernias should be repaired laparo-scopically if the resources are available and there is an experienced enough surgeon in laparoscopic procedures.

Apart from injecting local anaesthetic directly in the wound, are there any other procedures to improve post-operative pain in inguinal hernia repair?

Yes, one could perform an ileo-inguinal block. The landmark for needle insertion is 3 cm above and medial to the anterior superior iliac spine.

12. Femoral Hernia Repair

What is the commonest hernia in females?

Although the incidence of femoral hernia is higher in females compared with males, the incidence of inguinal hernia is still commoner in females.

Should all femoral hernias be repaired?

The general rule is that if a femoral hernia is present this should be repaired promptly for fear of strangulation. Although exceptions can be made in elderly, frail people where it has been picked up as an incidental finding.

What are the relations of the femoral canal?

- Anteriorly: inguinal ligament.
- Posteriorly: pectineal ligament.
- Medially: lacunar ligament.
- Laterally: femoral vein.

How would you repair a femoral hernia electively, using the Lockwood (low) approach?

A groin incision below medial half of the inguinal ligament. Layers are incised down to the sac of the hernia taking care to perform haemostasis on any saphenous vein tributaries. The hernial sac is exposed to the point where it emerges from beneath the inguinal ligament. The femoral vein will be close by and is protected with gentle retraction using a curved retractor. The sac is opened between two artery forceps to inspect the contents. If bowel contents are found they are assessed for viability. If viable, the bowel is returned to the abdomen and the neck of the sac transfixed and ligated with 2/0 vicryl. The sac is excised 1 cm distal to this ligature. The pectineal and inguinal ligaments are now opposed together such that the femoral canal is closed at the junction of the ligaments with the lacunar ligament (for approximately 1 cm laterally) without causing compression of the femoral vein. The suture used is usually nylon although any non-absorbable suture will suffice. Closure is performed in two layers (subcutaneous tissues and skin) with vicryl.

What approach would you use if a femoral hernia was strangulated in an emergency situation?

The best approach in these circumstances would be the McEvedy's (high) approach. The incision is made from 2–3 cm above the pubic tubercle, obliquely and laterally for 6–8 cm until the lateral extent of the rectus sheath. It is possible to assess the bowel, and if there is any doubt about its viability, the peritoneum can be opened over the neck of the hernia to allow resection of any gangrenous areas.

What key factors do you consider in determining the viability of the bowel at the time of femoral hernia surgery?

Healthy bowel is glistening, pinkish, peristalsing, with a pulsation in the mesenteric vessels. Gangrenous bowel may be black, green or purple bowel. If the bowel is of doubtful viability, but not frankly gangrenous, it can be covered with warmed normal saline packs and reassessed after a few minutes. Care is taken to examine any bowel caught at the neck of the hernia as these areas are very susceptible to ischaemic damage. In general, if there is any doubt about viability it is best to resect the bowel.

13. Laparoscopic Access

What techniques do you know of to induce a pneumoperitoneum?

The open (Hassan) method and the closed (Verres needle) method.

Describe one of these methods.

For the open (Hassan) method the patient should be tilted head down approximately 20–30 degrees (Trendelenberg's tilt). A small infraumbilical incision approximately 2 cm in length in the midline is made down to the linea alba. A J-shaped needle is inserted along with two stay sutures either side of the midline. These are used to lift the abdominal wall while the linea alba is incised under direct vision. Once the abdominal cavity is breeched a finger sweep is performed. A blunt ended trocar is inserted on a 10 mm laparoscopic port. This is done slowly with a screwing motion aiming towards the pelvis. Once positioned, a gas supply can be attached.

What settings would you use in insufflating the abdomen?

Between 2 and 4 l of carbon dioxide is delivered into the abdomen to an inflation pressure of 12–14 mmHg.

Are there any contraindications to performing laparoscopy?

Patients with generalised peritonitis, liver cirrhosis, clotting abnormalities and intestinal obstruction are generally considered absolute contraindications to laparoscopy. Relative contraindications would include ascites, significant organomegaly, gross obesity, pregnancy, abdominal aortic aneurysm (AAA), previous laparotomies and multiple adhesions.

What are the advantages to performing laparoscopic surgery over open surgery?

- Smaller incisions and as a result less trauma to tissues.
- Better cosmesis.
- Less post-operative pain requirements.
- Reduced incidence of wound complications.
- Quicker post-operative recovery with quicker mobilisation and less incidence of deep vain thrombosis (DVT).
- Less risk of blood contact transmission of human immunodeficiency virus (HIV) and Hepatitis B and C viruses.

Can you think of five complications or disadvantages of minimal access surgery?

- Lack of tactile feedback from tissues.
- Some procedures may have longer operating times.
- Malposition of trocar/Verres needle in the extraperitoneal space and insufflation of the wrong compartment.
- Risk of damage to great vessels, bowel with insertion of port sites and the Verres needle.
- Port site bleeding, herniation and infection.

14. Laparotomy

What do you understand by the term laparotomy?
Laparotomy refers to any surgery which involves opening the abdominal cavity.

What is the main advantage of a large midline laparotomy?
It allows for greater exposure of, and access to, the abdominal contents. This is particularly useful when operating on an acute abdomen with unknown underlying pathology.

You are performing a laparotomy and all appears normal on initial inspection. How do you proceed?
It is important to perform a consistent and methodical examination of the contents of the abdomen. A systematic approach is taken checking the viability of the major structures: liver and gall bladder, spleen, stomach, abdominal oesophagus, diaphragmatic hiatus, bile ducts, right kidney, duodenum, head of pancreas, transverse colon, body and tail of the pancreas, left kidney, superior mesenteric vessels, aorta, inferior mesenteric vessels, small bowel and its mesentry from the duodeno-jejunal flexure to the ileo-caecal valve, appendix, caecum, large bowel, rectum, ovaries, uterus, bladder, hernial orifices and the iliac vessels on either side.

In what circumstances when performing a laparotomy would you choose not to proceed with the operation once the peritoneum has been opened?
It would not be appropriate to proceed if florid carcinomatous disease or florid adhesions were found within the abdomen.

15. Appendicectomy

How would you prepare a patient for an appendicectomy?
Once the diagnosis of appendicitis is made, I would obtain appropriate informed consent, start intravenous fluids, and keep the patient nil by mouth. Cefuroxime and metronidazole can also be given intravenously. The patient is then taken to theatre and placed in the supine position. The entire abdomen should be cleaned and draped.

Where would you make your incision for an appendicectomy?

I would make a gridiron incision. This incision is at right angels to a line joining the anterior superior iliac spine to the umbilicus and passes through McBurney's point (a point one third of the way from the anterior superior iliac spine to the umbilicus).

What layers are traversed in such an incision?

- Skin.
- Fat.
- Scarpa's fascia.
- Fat.
- External oblique aponeurosis.
- Internal oblique.
- Transversus abdominis.
- Transversalis fascia and peritoneum which are fused.

How do you locate the appendix?

By finding the caecum and following the taenia to the base of the appendix.

How would you remove the appendix?

The mesoappendix is clamped with artery forcep and ligated 2/0 vicryl. A seromuscular purse-string suture is placed around the base of the appendix using 2/0 vicryl. The base of the appendix is crushed with a haemostat and then replaced with a clamp 5 mm further up the appendix. The crushed base of the appendix is ligated with a 0 vicryl tie. A blade is used to cut the appendix off below the haemostat. The appendix stump is then buried in the bowel wall and secured with the previously placed purse-string suture.

What would you do if the appendix was normal?

Remove it for histological examination and examine for other pathology in the right iliac fossa, such as: a carcinoid tumour of the appendix, inflammation or cancer of the caecum, mesenteric adenitis, a Meckel's diverticulum, iliac aneurysm and the cysts in the right ovary.

What are the complications of an appendicectomy?

- Scars.
- Reactive haemorrhage.
- Wound infection.
- Abscess.
- Increase incidence of right inguinal hernia.

16. Splenectomy

What are the functions of the spleen?

The spleen is a major organ of the reticulo-endothelial system and has the flowing functions:

- Immune: antigen processing, opsonin production and immunoglobulin M (IgM) production.
- Removal of waste: removal of old and defective platelets, and removal of red blood cells.
- Filtration: macrophages are predominantly responsible for destroying cellular and non-cellular materials, such as bacteria and foreign materials.
- Redistribution of iron: cells within the spleen return the iron from killed red blood cells to the plasma.
- Haemopoiesis: in the foetus-only states.

Can you think of some causes of splenomegaly?

- Infective: malaria, leishmaniasis, tuberculosis, HIV, cytomegalovirus (CMV) and Epstein–Barr virus (EBV).
- Splenic congestion: portal hypertension (any cause), alcoholic liver disease and cirrhosis.
- Cellular proliferation: haemolytic anaemias and myeloproliferative disorders.
- Deficiencies: severe iron deficiency and pernicious anaemia.
- Auto-immune: rheumatiod arthritis (Felty's syndrome) and systemic lupus erythematosus (SLE).

What important relations of the spleen can be damaged in performing splenectomy?

- Posteriorly: diaphragm and 9–11th ribs.
- Anteriorly: stomach.
- Medially: left kidney and the tail of the pancreas.
- Inferiorly: splenic flexure of the colon.

What vessels are carried in the lieno-renal and gastro-splenic ligaments?

The gastro-splenic ligament, from the greater curvature of the stomach to the spleen, carries the left gastro-epiploic vessels and the short gastrics. The lieno-renal ligament runs from the posterior abdominal wall to the spleen and carries the splenic vessels.

Can you give two medical indications for splenectomy?

- Auto-immune haemolysis/thrombocytopaenia.
- Hereditary sphaerocytosis and elliptocytosis.

What are the principles in performing an emergency splenectomy?

This is usually performed for a ruptured spleens secondary to trauma. An upper midline abdominal incision is used which may be extended to the left costal margin. Two large suction catheters are kept to hand in case of massive bleeding. Once the peritoneal cavity is open an excessive blood is suctioned off. Large packs are placed in the left upper quadrant if bleeding is still not controlled. The spleen is mobilised forward into the wound cavity by cutting free the attachment of the left limb of the lieno-renal ligament (this is often achievable with the use of fingers alone in ruptured spleens). The vascular pedicle on the undersurface of the spleen is compressed to control haemorrhage. This is done initially with finger and thumb until access is sufficient to place a large clamp. Once the bleeding is controlled excess blood is removed and the spleen inspected. The lesser sac is entered through the greater omentum and any adhesions between the spleen and stomach/pancreas divided. The splenic artery is identified at the top of the pancreas tied off. The spleen is freed from the splenic flexure and diaphragm the anterior leaf of the gastro-splenic ligament incised. The short gastric vessels are tied off taking care not to inadvertently tie part of the stomach. There should now be adequate access to the vascular pedicle of the spleen to tie it off. The vessels at the pedicle of the spleen (splenic artery and vein) are double clamoed taking care not to injure the tail of the pancreas. The spleen can now be removed. The operative field is reassessed and checked for haemostasis. A drain is left in the splenic bed and the abdomen closured in layers.

What risks are present to the asplenic patient and what measures are taken to reduce these?

With the spleen removed the patient is at risk of over-whelming infection because encapsulated bacteria are normally destroyed by the spleen. Common pathogens include *Streptococcus pneumonia*, *Neisseria meningitidis* and *Haemophilus influenzae*. Patients are at risk of severe malaria if exposed, and animal and tick bites may be dangerous. Patients are educated to the potential risks and measures they must take in suspected infections and are given with vaccinations against the aforementioned bacteria. Most patients are given 500-mg penicillin once a day for life, although this protocol varies from institute to institute.

17. Cholecystectomy

What are the indications for performing a cholecystectomy?

- Gallstones.
- Carcinoma of the gall bladder.

What are the contraindications to performing a laparoscopic cholecystectomy?
- Cirrhosis with portal hypertension.
- Common bile duct stones.
- Pregnancy.
- Morbid obesity.
- Previous abdominal surgery (adhesions and difficult laparoscopic access).
- Acute cholecystitis.

In the right hands (e.g. those of hepato-pancreatico-biliary surgeons), laparoscopic surgery can be performed within 4 weeks of diagnosis of acute cholecystitis, and may even be performed in the presence of cirrhosis. However, in acute cholecystitis, severe inflammatory changes may obscure the normal anatomy so that the laparoscopic technique may not be suitable.

In obtaining consent for laparoscopic cholecystectomy, what important risks should be explained to the patient?
- Risk of injury to the common bile duct.
- Possibility of jaundice.
- Infection.
- Pain.
- Haemorrhage.
- Possibility of converting to an open procedure.

In performing laparoscopic cholecystectomy how many ports will you use?
Four ports: umbilical, epigastric, right lateral and one other variable port.

Can you describe the landmarks for the insertion of these ports?
- Umbilical port: a 10-mm port placed in the infraumbilical position (the camera is usually placed in this port).
- Epigastric port: a 10-mm port placed just right of the midline 4–6 cm below the xiphisternum (dissection and diathermy is carried out in the formation of this port).
- Right lateral port: a 5-mm port placed in the right midquadrant lateral to the midclavicular line (retraction of the gall bladder is carried out using a right lateral port).
- Fourth variable port: a 5-mm port in the right upper quadrant, midclavicular line.

What is Calot's triangle and why is it important to identify?

Calot's triangle is a triangle made up of the inferior surface of the liver, the common hepatic duct and the cystic duct. It contains the cystic artery (a branch of the right hepatic artery) and the cystic node. This triangle must be identified and dissected so that the cystic artery and duct can be clearly identified and divided.

How can you ensure that you are dividing the cystic artery and not the right hepatic artery?

By following the path of the cystic artery the gall bladder wall which it supplies.

When would you perform an intra-operative cholangiogram?

There are various bodies of opinion. Some surgeons prefer to perform it routinely to demarcate the anatomy of the biliary tree. Others hold that it be performed only when there is clinical, biochemical and ultrasound evidence of gallstones in the common bile duct. Finally, there are those who believe that it should never be performed intra-operatively because preoperative endoscopic retrograde cholangio-pancreatography (ERCP) can confirm the absence of stones on the common bile duct.

Can you give five indications for ERCP?

- Obstructive jaundice with dilated common bile duct.
- Recurrent cholangitis.
- Recurrent pancreatitis.
- Assessment of common bile duct prior to laparoscopic cholecystectomy.
- Palliative or preoperative stenting of malignant biliary stricture.

18. Nephrectomy

Can you summarise briefly the anatomical relations of the kidneys?

- Posteriorly (both kidneys): diaphragm, quadratus lumborum, psoas major muscle, transversus abdominis, 12th rib, subcostal nerve, ileo-hypogastric nerve and ileo-inguinal nerve.
- Anteriorly
  Left kidney: stomach, pancreas, spleen and descending colon.
  Right kidney: liver, second part of the duodenum and ascending colon.
- Medially (both kidneys): hilar structures (renal vein, renal artery, ureter and lymphatics).

Describe the anatomical layers you would traverse in a posterior approach to the kidney.

- Skin.
- Subcutaneous fat.
- Deep fascia.
- External oblique/latissimus dorsi muscle.
- Internal oblique muscle.
- Transversus abdominis and quadratus lumborum.
- Paranephric fat.
- Ileoinguinal and ileohypogastric nerves.
- Posterior surface of Gerota's fascia.
- Perinephric fat.
- Renal capsule.

What is the difference between a radical and simple nephrectomy?

A simple nephrectomy involves simple removal of the kidney, where as radical surgery involves excision of the kidney along with Gerota's fascia, the adrenal gland and local lymph nodes. The radical technique has shown to be superior in terms of survival rates, when performed for localised renal cancer.

What are the indications for nephron-sparing surgery?

Essentially, any situation which may result in renal insufficiency, e.g. non-functioning contralateral kidney and bilateral small tumour.

Renal cell carcinomas may present with renal vein or inferior vena cava involvement. What is the surgical significance of this?

Control above and below the thrombus must be achieved as well as control of the contralateral renal vein in order to prevent further spread of the malignancy.

19. Hemicolectomy

Can you name three indications for performing a right hemicolectomy?

- Carcinoma of the caecum.
- Carcinoma of the appendix.
- Crohn's disease of the right colon.

What incision would you make in performing a right hemicolectomy?

A midline or right paramedian incision.

What structures are at risk in a right hemicolectomy?

- Right ureter.
- Pancreas.
- Duodenum.
- Right gonadal vessels.

Which arteries are divided in performing a right hemicolectomy?

- Ileo-colic artery.
- Right colic artery.
- Right branch of the middle colic artery.

Where would you divide these vessels?

The vessels are divided as close to their origin as possible, i.e. the superior mesenteric artery. This is performed to facilitate good surgical clearance, in cases of carcinoma, and also for adequate mobilisation of the two ends left to be anastomosed. In cases of benign disease, the vessels may be divided in the middle of the mesentery when only a limited resection is required.

Where should the proximal resection margin be?

Usually the proximal margin includes 20 cm of terminal ileum. However, this may increase to involve more small bowel in cases affecting the small bowel and the right side of the colon, e.g. Crohn's disease.

20. Endoscopy

Give three indications for an endoscopic examination of the oesophagus and upper gastrointestinal tract?

- Upper gastrointestinal bleed.
- Dysphagia not explained by a neurological disease.
- Pain on swallowing.

How would you prepare a patient for this type of endoscopy?

Informed consent would need to be obtained from the patient. Any dentures should be removed and the patient should be starved for

5 hours. In an emergency situation a nasogastric tube can be used to empty the stomach. Adequate cardiovascular monitoring should be employed, i.e. a pulse oximeter and electrocardiography (ECG). Intravenous access is obtained. The pharynx should be sprayed with lignocaine solution. The patient is positioned on the left side with the hips and knees flexed. Controlled sedation may be achieved with midazolam ensuring that reversal agents are close to hand.

How far is it from the mouth to the cricopharyngeal sphincter and cardia of the stomach?
- Cricopharyngeal sphincter: 16 cm.
- Cardia: 40 cm.

What are the complications of an upper gastrointestinal endoscopy?
- Perforation of the oesophagus, stomach or duodenum.
- Mediastinitis.
- Bleeding.

What preparation would a patient require for flexible sigmoidoscopy and colonoscopy?
A phosphate enema for flexible sigmoidoscopy and a full-bowel preparation for colonoscopy.

21. Abdominal Aortic Aneurysm Repair

Can give three indications for AAA repair?
- Aneurysm rupture.
- Aneurysm size >5.5 cm.
- A tender aneurysm.

Describe the preoperative preparations for an elective repair.
Appropriate preoperative investigations should be carried out (full blood count (FBC), urea and electrolytes (U&E), coagulation screen, chest X-ray (CXR) and ECG). In addition, some patients may require arterial blood gases, respiratory function tests, echocardiogram, and a carotid duplex. At least 6 units of blood, 2 units of fresh frozen plasma and 2 pools of platelets should be cross-matched. Informed consent must be obtained from the patient. A central venous pressure (CVP) line, arterial line and urinary catheter will need to be inserted preoperatively. The patient is laid supine and the abdomen cleaned and draped

from xiphisternum to both groins. Broad-spectrum intravenous antibiotics are given on induction.

Describe briefly the approach to the abdominal aorta.

A long midline incision (from xiphisternum to the pubis) skirting the umbilicus is used. The small bowel is retracted to the right and packed in a large swab. The peritoneum over the aorta is then divided to expose the aneurysm neck.

How does the mortality of elective repair compare to emergency repair?

Elective should be <5%. Emergency repair is associated with mortalities of >40%.

What are the common causes of death following AAA repair?

- Myocardial infarction.
- Renal failure.
- Respiratory complications.

22. Abscess

What is an abscess?
A localised collection of pus.

What antibiotics should be started for an abscess?
Antibiotics play no part in the initial management of abscesses. The abscess requires surgical drainage.

What are the different types of anal abscess?
- Perianal.
- Intersphincteric.
- Supralevator.
- Ischiorectal.
- Intermuscular.

How would you drain an anal abscess?
After obtaining appropriate informed consent, with the patient anaesthetised and in the lithotomy position, an incision is made over the abscess removing any dead tissue. The cavity is curretted and washed out with saline and betadine. A drain is then placed into the cavity.

23. Sebaceous Cyst

What are the characteristics of a sebaceous cyst?
A sebaceous cyst is a round, smooth and firm to soft swelling attached to the skin. A punctum is usually present.

What is Gardner's syndrome?
Multiple cysts in association with intestinal polyposis, osteomas and desmoid tumours.

What local anaesthetics might you use?
Lignocaine, prilocaine or bubivicane.

What are the safe doses of these local anaesthetics?
- Bubivicane: 2 mg/kg.
- Lignocaine: 3 mg/kg.
- Lignocaine with adrenaline 1 in 250,000: 6 mg/kg.
- Prilocaine: 10 mg/kg.

When must you not use adrenaline?

When injecting a digit or appendage.

How would you remove the cyst?

After obtaining appropriate informed consent, an elliptical incision is made around the punctum of the cyst along Langer's lines. The cyst is then dissected out taking care not to rupture it. If the cyst is punctured the wound should be washed out with normal saline.

What would you do with the specimen if you were confident it was a sebaceous cyst?

I would make sure to send it to the pathologist for histological confirmation.

24. Nail Excision

What procedure do you know for the treatment of in growing toenails?

Zadek's operation – radical resection of the nail bed.

When should you not perform this operation?

This should not be performed in the presence of infection or peripheral vascular disease.

What anaesthetic technique would you use?

A local ring block with lignocaine using a digital tourniquet. Adrenaline would not be used.

How would you perform the operation?

After obtaining informed consent, and performing the anaesthetic technique described above, the lower leg would be cleaned and draped. The nail would be removed from the nail bed using a MacDonald's elevator. A skin flap would then be raised at the proximal end of the nail by making two incisions from both corners of the nail extending to the distal skin crease. The skin flap would then be retracted to clear the germinal matrix of the nail. At each side a block of the nail bed would be removed back to the insertion of the extensor tendon. The skin incisions would then be closed and the wound dressed with a non-absorbent dressing and the tourniquet released.

What advise would you give the patient?

The patient should be advised to elevate the leg for 1 day and weight bare as pain allowed. The dressing and sutures would be removed after 12 days.

25. Lymph Node Biopsy

Where are common sites for lymph node biopsies?
Groin, axilla and neck.

What anaesthetic would you use?
General anaesthetic as dissection is usually harder than anticipated.

How would you prepare the patient for surgery?
Appropriate informed consent and the lymph node that is to be biopsied is marked.

How would you perform an excision lymph node biopsy?
Position the patient appropriately, clean and drape the biopsy site. An incision is made over the lymph node along Langer's lines. The lymph node is dissected from the surrounding tissue handling the lymph gland very gently. The lymph node is removed gently to achieve haemostasis.

What would you do with the specimen?
Divide the lymph node into two sending it for histology and microbiology.

What are the complications of lymph mode biopsies?
- Haematoma.
- Infection (especially with groin dissection).
- Damage to local structures (e.g. nerves in neck dissections).

26. Tru-cut Biopsy

How would you prepare a patient for a Tru-cut biopsy of a tumour?
After explaining the procedure to the patient I would clearly identify the lesion and clean the area over the lesion.

How would you anaesthetise the area?
I would infiltrate the skin over the lesion with 1% lignocaine and continue injecting deeper until I had entered the tumour.

How would you take the biopsy?
A small incision would be made over the lesion. The tumour would be fixed with one hand and the inner needle of the Tru-cut needle

pushed into the tumour. The outer sheath of the needle is then fully advanced. The whole Tru-cut needle would then be removed with the biopsy sample.

What would you do if the sample was not satisfactory?

Repeat the procedure trying to obtain adequate tissue.

What would you do with the biopsy?

Place the biopsy specimen in a labelled specimen pot containing formaldehyde and send the specimen for histology after contacting the laboratory.

27. Approach to Hip

Name one common approach to the hip joint?
The direct lateral approach (Hardinge approach).

Briefly describe how you would perform this approach?
Informed consent is taken from the patient preoperatively taking care to ensure that the correct hip is marked for operation. In theatre, the patient is positioned laterally with the affected hip uppermost. A longitudinal incision is made beginning 10 to 15 cm below the greater trochanter, curving 30° posteriorly, from the tip of the greater trochanter to a point which cuts a line subtended vertically down from the anterior superior iliac spine. Fascia lata is incised over the midpoint of the trochanter distally in the line of the femur and proximally the incision divides superficial and deep layers of the fascia lata. The enclosed gluteus maximus is cut in the line of its fibres. The tendon of gluteus medius is cut from its attachment to the greater trochanter and the incision extended through vastus lateralis onto the anterior aspect of the femur. The capsule of the hip joint is now in view and can be incised to open the joint.

Which nerve is particularly at risk in this approach?
The superior gluteal nerve.

What would be the clinical consequences of division of the superior gluteal nerve?
This nerve supplies the gluteus medius and minimus muscles. Damage to this nerve, therefore, results in loss of hip abduction and a Trendelenberg gait.

What manoeuvre is performed with the leg to expose the fractured femoral neck?
Adduction and external rotation.

What structures are at risk in a posterior approach to the hip?
The sciatic nerve.

What is a Smith–Petterson approach?
This is an anterior approach to the hip joint which exploits the internervous plane between sartorius (femoral nerve) and tensor fascia lata (superior gluteal nerve). It is used in paediatric orthopaedics to correct congenital dislocation of the hip.

28. Lower Limb Amputations

Which amputation offers the patient the best chance of walking again, below knee or above knee?

Below knee. The above knee amputation, however, has a higher primary healing rate.

Why is it important to use prophylactic antibiotics in amputation surgery?

Presence of necrotic tissue encourages proliferation of *Clostridium perfringens*, therefore the risk of gas gangrene is high.

Describe how you would plan the flaps and level of bone division for an above knee amputation?

Equal anterior and posterior flaps are marked. Bony division must allow at least 15 cm clearance from the level of the knee joint.

How would you proceed?

The skin and fascia are divided in line with flaps already marked. Muscle groups are divided next with neurovascular bundles ligated as one proceeds. A rougine is then used to strip the periosteum from the femur at the anticipated level of trans-section. This must be at least 5 cm proximal to where muscle groups were divided. The femur is divided and the edges smoothened using a file. The muscles, fascia and skin are then approximated in layers. A Redivac drain is laid in one of the deeper layers, brought out laterally and left unsutured.

Why is it important to commence physiotherapy as early as possible?

This prevents flexion contractures and optimises chances of regaining mobility with a prosthesis.

29. Approach to Knee

What common approaches to the knee are you aware of?

The anteromedial approach which is used in total knee replacement surgery.

Describe this approach briefly.

A longitudinal incision is made beginning at the medial border of the quadriceps tendon 7–10 cm proximal to the patella and extending inferiorly. The incision curved to the medial aspect of the patella then returns to the midline inferiorly to end at the tibial tuberosity. The capsule of the knee is exposed by dividing fascia and dissecting between the vastus medialis muscle and the quadriceps tendon. The capsule is incised to gain access to the knee joint. The patella is reflected laterally and the knee flexed to obtain the best view.

What neurovascular structures are at risk?
- The saphenous nerve and the great saphenous vein.
- The geniculate vessels which anastomose around the knee.

Is the posterior longitudinal ligament routinely sacrificed in a knee replacement?
The posterior cruciate is preserved or sacrificed according to the type of knee replacement being performed. Posterior cruciate deficient knees a constrained design of tibial insert.

What is the approximate incidence of deep vein thrombosis in knee surgery?
Approximately 75%. This can be reduced with good hydration, early mobilisation, and the use of graded elastic compression stockings or intermittent pneumatic calf compression. Heparin prophylaxis with low molecular weight drugs like heparin are also employed.

30. Exposure of Vessels

Can you recall three indications for exposure of the brachial artery?
- To carry out an embolectomy.
- Exploration of the artery following trauma, e.g. supracondylar fracture of the humerus.
- To obtain access for endovascular approaches.

How would you expose the artery?
The artery lies on the medial aspect of the upper arm covered by the tendon of biceps. A vertical S-shaped ("lazy S") incision is made in the antecubital fossa. The biceps tendon is then partially divided to locate the artery between biceps and brachialis. The median nerve lies next to the artery and must be identified and preserved.

What surface land marks are used to locate the femoral artery?
The artery lies at the midinguinal point. This is located midway on a line drawn between the pubic symphysis and the anterior superior iliac spine.

What structures are encountered during exposure of the common femoral artery?

The incision over the artery is deepened by cutting through subcutaneous fat, staying medial to sartorius. Lymph nodes are usually found in the fat. The femoral sheath is divided to expose the artery. The inguinal ligament lies superiorly and may need to be divided to improve proximal exposure, the femoral vein lies medial to the artery and the femoral nerve lies deep and lateral to the artery.

Can you name some of the complications associated with the groin incision used?

- Wound infection.
- Haematoma.
- Lymphocoele/persistent lymph leak.
- Flap necrosis.
- Scarring.

31. Varicose Veins

What is the prevalence of varicose veins in the general population?

Approximately 2%.

Can you name a few secondary causes of varicosities?

- Valvular damage due to previous deep vein thrombosis.
- Pregnancy.
- Pelvic tumour.
- Congenital valvular agenesis.

How is the patient positioned on the table for long saphenous varicose vein surgery?

The patient is laid supine with 30 degrees head down tilt (Trendelenberg's position). The legs should be straight and abducted with the feet resting on the edges of a long board across lower end of table.

What incision would you use to locate the saphenofemoral junction in the groin?

A 5-cm long incision parallel to the inguinal ligament and along the groin crease is used. It should be centred 2.5 cm below and lateral to the pubic tubercle.

How would you proceed once the incision is made?

The incision is deepened and fatty tissues swept away using a swab until the long saphenous vein and its tributaries are identified. All tributaries are divided between clips and ligated. The vein is followed through the cribriform fascia to confirm its junction with the femoral vein. It is then clipped and divided. A double tie is used to ligate the proximal end flush with the femoral vein.

How would you strip the long saphenous vein?

A small incision is made in the vein allowing passage of a long stripper to below the knee. The distal tip of the stripper is cut down onto and it is then brought out of the vein. A 1-cm olive is applied to the tip of the stripper. A handle is then attached to the proximal end of the stripper and, with gentle traction along the long axis of the leg, the stripper is pulled up through the thigh.

32. Carpal Tunnel Decompression

What are the signs and symptoms of carpal tunnel syndrome?

Pain and parasthesia in the distribution of the median nerve on the radial side of the hand with preserved sensation over the thenar eminence. The patient complains of waking at night with burning pain, numbness or tingling in the hand. This is classically relieved by hanging their arm out of bed or shaking it. Symptoms may be exacerbated by pressure over the carpal tunnel, prolonged wrist flexion (Phalen's test) and Tinel's sign may be positive at the wrist.

What are the risk factors for carpal tunnel syndrome?

- Obesity.
- Diabetes mellitus.
- Thyroid dysfunction.
- Rheumatoid arthritis.
- Pregnancy.
- Ganglion.
- Lipoma.
- Repetitive use of vibrating tools.
- Trauma (e.g. fractures of distal radius).
- Tight bandaging/plaster immobilisation.
- Wrist immobilisation in extreme flexion following fracture manipulation.

What other conditions should be excluded and what investigations would you perform to establish a diagnosis?

Symptoms mimic a cervical spondylosis (non-specific degeneration of the spine) at C6/C7. Commonly, cervical spine X-rays will show degenerative changes in this age group causing confusion. Nerve conduction studies, particularly of sensory nerve velocities, are most sensitive, although they may still be apparently normal. Comparison with the ulnar nerve velocities may be helpful.

Are there any other investigations that can be used to help confirm the diagnosis?

A carpal tunnel series of X-rays may show bony impingement of the tunnel. Magnetic resonance imaging (MRI) may reveal a space occupying soft tissue lesion in the tunnel.

What are the treatment options for carpal tunnel syndrome?

Non-operative management, e.g. hydrocortisone injection into the carpal tunnel and splintage may be employed. In addition, other correctable causes should be investigated and treated including thyroid disorders and diabetes. Surgical management is by carpal tunnel decompression.

What are the surgical options for carpal tunnel syndrome?

- Open division of the deep transverse carpal ligament.
- Closed division of the deep transverse carpal ligament.

What is the predicted outcome of carpal tunnel decompression?

Symptoms improve in at least 85% of patients and thenar muscle atrophy may also resolve.

Describe the surgical approach to open carpal tunnel decompression.

The procedure can be performed under general, regional or local anaesthesia, with or without tourniquet control. A longitudinal gently curved incision is made parallel to the thenar skin crease extending proximally to the distal wrist crease. The incision should lie on the ulnar side of the middle finger axis in the line of palmaris longus. Layers are incised to expose the flexor retinaculum. A small incision is made in the flexor retinaculum so that a blunt dissector can be placed beneath the ligament. The blunt dissector can be manipulated to loosen any scar tissue from the deep surface of the flexor retinaculum. Using an instrument, such as a MacDonald's, to protect the median nerve the flexor retinaculum is incised longitudinally. The skin is with interrupted non-absorbable sutures and dressed liberally with absorbent non-constrictive dressings.

What are the possible complications of carpal tunnel surgery?

- Infection.
- Haemorrhage.
- Nerve damage: to the median nerve itself, of the recurrent motor branch or of the palmar cutaneous branch.

33. Fasciotomies

What do you understand by the term compartment syndrome?

Raised pressure in an unyielding osseofascial compartment causes compression of the enclosed structures. It most commonly occurs in the limbs.

How does compartment syndrome arise?

It can be acute due to fractures and associated soft-tissue injury, crush injury, or reperfusion injury following a revascularisation procedure. It may also be chronic, especially following exercise. Following an injury, fracture haematoma and soft tissue oedema may exceed the potential space available in the compartment resulting in increased pressure. Sustained elevation of pressure leads to diminished capillary perfusion to a level below that necessary for tissue viability. This results in irreversible muscle and nerve damage within hours in the acute situation.

What would you make you suspicious of a compartment syndrome in a limb?

The history gives the first clues, e.g. a crush injury, increases index of suspicion. The patient will complain of pain disproportionate to the injury and which is non-responsive to analgesia. Pain exacerbated by passive stretch of the muscles in the compartment is particularly worrying. There may also be paraesthesia and paralysis of the affected compartment. Compartment syndrome differs from an acutely ischaemic limb because the ischaemic damage is due to diminished capillary perfusion rather than arterial perfusion. Presence of pulses, therefore, does not exclude a compartment syndrome.

Is there any investigation you could do to help diagnose compartment syndrome?

Intra-compartmental pressure measurement. Compartmental pressures of $>40\,\text{mmHg}$, or $\text{BP}_{\text{diastolic}} - \text{Pres}_{\text{cmpt}} <30\,\text{mmHg}$, are indicative of impending compartment syndrome.

What is the principle of management?

Careful attention to medical sequelae and surgical decompression of the affected compartment.

How would you perform a fasciotomy for decompression of the compartments of the lower leg?

The anterior and lateral compartments are decompressed through a full-length anterolateral skin incision 2 cm anterior to the fibula from just proximal to the ankle to the level of the tibial tubersosity. The underlying fascia is divided and subcutaneous dissection allows decompression of the lateral compartment. The superficial branch of the peroneal nerve is identified and protected. Superficial and deep posterior compartments are approached via a longitudinal incision just medial to the posteromedial border of the tibia. The deep fascia is divided from tibial tuberosity to 5 cm proximal to the medial malleolus. Necrosed muscle is excised and staged debridement is necessary before closure is considered.

What are the possible medical sequelae of acute compartment syndrome?

- Rhabdomyolysis.
- Hyperkalaemia.
- Acidosis.
- Myoglobinuria.
- Acute tubular necrosis.

34. Vascular Anastomosis

What suture materials are used for vascular anastomosis?

Synthetic, non-absorbable sutures such as polypropelene.

Can you name two common materials that vascular grafts are constructed from?

Polytetrafluoroethylene (PTFE) and Dacron.

What are the principles of anastomosis?

The anastomosis must be tension-free and there should not be a large size mismatch between vessels or vessel and graft. Systemic heparin should be administered before anastomosis to reduce thrombogenicity of vessel/graft surfaces. The intima of the vessel should not be damaged (e.g. do not grasp intima with forceps) and the anastomosis should be water-tight.

How is the risk of an intimal flap developing inside the anastomosed vessel kept to a minimum?

Sutures placed in the downstream end of the anastomosis must be inserted from inside the vessel to out. This ensures that the intima is "tacked" down.

Can you think of any techniques used to overcome the problem of graft to vessel size mismatch?

Smaller grafts can be anastomosed end to side with the vessel. The end of the graft to be anastomosed can be cut at an angle to increase the size interface. A segment of vein can be used to construct a Miller's cuff or St Mary's Boot in order to provide a wider interface between large graft (e.g. 8 mm PTFE) and small crural vessel in femoro-distal bypass.

Applied Physiology

CELLULAR PHYSIOLOGY

FLUIDS AND ELECTROLYTES

RENAL PHYSIOLOGY

GASTROINTESTINAL PHYSIOLOGY

ENDOCRINE PHYSIOLOGY

VASCULAR PHYSIOLOGY

CARDIAC PHYSIOLOGY

RESPIRATORY PHYSIOLOGY

1. Membranes

What is the main function of the cell membrane?
To control the entry and exit of molecules from the cell and so regulate the intracellular environment.

Describe the basic structure of a cell membrane.
The cell membrane consists of a continuous lipid bilayer studded with protein molecules.

How does this structure allow control of the movement of molecules into and out of the cell?
The lipid bilayer has hydrophilic groups facing outwards while hydrophobic groups face each other across the middle. Most large water-soluble molecules, charged molecules and ions cannot cross the lipid barrier. Size, charge and water-solubility all decrease the ability of a molecule crossing the fatty membrane. These substances depend on the membrane proteins for their entry and exit from the cell. These proteins can act as channels sensitive to voltage or ligand-binding or as energy-dependent pumps. Fat-soluble substances like oxygen and carbon dioxide can cross easily as can water.

What is the overall charge of the outer surface of the cell membrane?
Negative.

What part of the membrane structure is responsible for this negative charge?
The cell has a "glycocalyx" formed by membrane carbohydrates, which are negatively charged. These carbohydrates also act as receptor substrates and can bind to carbohydrates on other cells.

2. Ion Channels

What is the basic structure of an ion channel?
They are proteins, which form tubular structures with a central pore which traverses the cell membrane and can allow communication between the extracellular fluid and the intracellular compartment.

Are they simple pores?

No, they are selectively permeable to specific ions and can be opened and closed.

What would be the consequences for nerve conduction if they were simple pores?

If they were open all the time there could be no electrical potential across the cell membrane and cells would be isoelectric with the extracellular environment. The lack of ion gradient would remove the power source for the action potential to be generated when ion channels open and so nerve conduction would not be possible.

What features of an ion channels make it selective for sodium or potassium ions?

This is determined by the pore diameter and the charge within the channel. A sodium selective channel is highly charged and narrow. In a charged environment ions dehydrate and the dehydrated Na^+ ion is smaller than dehydrated K^+ and so can selectively pass through. The potassium selective channel is less charged so the ions are hydrated, a hydrated K^+ ion is smaller than hydrated Na^+ and the pore is the right size to let the hydrated K^+ through.

How can mechanisms of channel gating be classified? Please give examples.

Channels can be voltage or ligand gating. An example of a voltage-gated channel is the Na^+ channel in the membrane of a nerve fibre where the gate is strongly shut when the intracellular charge is negative. If the cell becomes less negative the gate opens allowing Na^+ ions to flood in and generate the action potential. An example of a ligand-gated channel is the acetylcholine receptor at the neuromuscular junction. Acetylcholine interacts with the channel leading to a conformational change which opens the central pore to allow Na^+ ion to flood into the cell.

3. Receptors

What is a receptor?

The specific molecular site to which a pharmacological agent binds and mediates its effect.

Explain how binding to a receptor can lead to a cellular response.

A receptor has two components, the binding part which protrudes from the cell membrane and an ionophore component which passes through the membrane to the intracellular compartment. The ionophore can be an enzyme or an ion channel. In the case of an ion channel, binding of a ligand leads to the opening of a gate and influx or efflux of ions as is the case at the neuromuscular junction when acetylcholine binds. Enzyme-linked receptors alter the metabolic activity of the cell often via second messengers. Cyclic adenosine monophosphate (AMP) production by adenyl cyclase is mediated by ligand-binding followed by G-protein activation. Protein kinases can lead to altered gene expression in the nucleus. In general, enzyme-linked receptors lead to slow, prolonged changes in cell activity and ion channels to rapid, short-lived responses to receptor-binding.

What is a neurotransmitter?

A chemical which binds to a receptor and leads to an effect on synapse function in nerve conduction.

Give an example of an excitatory and inhibitory neurotransmitter.

Acetylcholine is an excitatory neurotransmitter at muscarinic receptors while gamma-amino-butyric acid (GABA) is the main inhibitory neurotransmitter in the brain.

When is manipulation of the acetylcholine receptor of interest to the surgeon?

Blocking transmission at the neuro-muscular junction by blocking the acetylcholine receptor with a muscle relaxant paralyses the patient.

How do patients with myasthenia gravis behave differently to muscle relaxants?

They are resistant to depolarising agents like suxamethonium but more sensitive to non-depolarising agents such as atracurium.

4. Action Potentials

Draw and describe a neuronal action potential.

A typical neuronal action potential is shown in Figure 4. There are three phases to an action potential:

1. Resting phase – negative charge maintained by $Na^+/K^+/ATPase$.
2. Depolarisation phase – after a threshold is reached Na^+ channels open and the cell becomes more positively charged and actually overshoots beyond neutral.

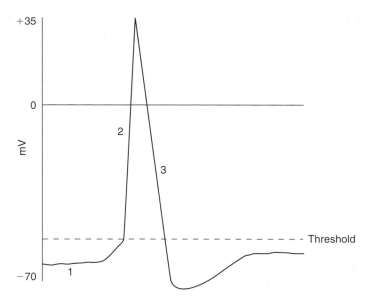

Figure 4 Neuronal action potential.

3. Repolarisation phase – Na^+ channels close and K^+ channels open leading to the cell returning to a negative state. Again there is overshoot and the cell become hyperpolarised.

Draw and describe a typical cardiac action potential.

A typical cardiac action potential is shown in Figure 5. There are four phases to the cardiac action potential:

1. Depolarisation and overshoot due to Na^+ channels opening.
2. Repolarisation as Na^+ channels shut.
3. Plateau phase as Ca^{2+} enter.

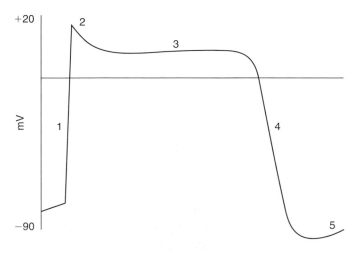

Figure 5 Cardiac action potential.

4. Repolarisation as K$^+$ effluxes.
5. Slow upward drift due to Na$^+$ entry, cell is refractory during this period.

Draw and describe the action potential in the sino-atrial node.

A typical sino-atrial nodal action potential is shown in Figure 6. There are three phases to the nodal action potential:

1. Upwards drift due to leak of Na$^+$ ions into the cell.
2. When threshold of -40 mV reached rapid entry of Ca^{2+} ions occurs.
3. Repolarisation due to K$^+$ efflux.

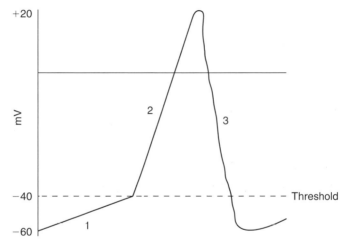

Figure 6 Sino-atrial nodal action potential.

5. Distribution of Body Water

What are the different fluid compartments of the body?

Total body water accounts for 50–70% of body weight. It is distributed into intracellular fluid (30–40% of body weight) and extracellular fluid (ECF) (20% of body weight). ECF is further divided into interstitial fluid (15% of body weight) and intravascular fluid (5% of body weight). The interstitial compartment increases in size and accounts for third-space fluid that accumulates after an operation, burn, trauma or severe illness.

How do you determine the size of the fluid compartments?

Total body water comprises approximately two-thirds of body weight. Of this, two-thirds is intracellular and one-third is extracellular. Of the extracellular compartment, two-thirds is interstitial and one-third is intravascular. However, there is a higher percentage of water in the young, thin and men, and a lower percentage in the elderly, obese and women.

What is meant by osmolarity and osmolality?

Osmolarity is a measure of concentration per litre of solution. Osmolality is a measure of concentration per kilogram of solvent. Osmolality of plasma is maintained at 280–305 mosmol/kg. It may be estimated by

$$mosmol/kg = glucose + urea + (2 \times sodium) \ (mmol/l).$$

How do intravenous fluids distribute when infused into the body?

Normal saline rapidly distributes across the entire extravascular compartment, which is four times as large as the intravascular compartment. So, of 1000 ml of normal saline, only 250 ml would remain in the intravascular compartment. Five per cent dextrose distributes across both intracellular and extracellular compartments. The intravascular compartment represents only 5/40ths of the fluid compartments as a whole. So, only 8% or 80 ml of 5% dextrose would remain in the intravascular compartment.

What are the common causes of water excess?

- The infusion of 5% dextrose.
- Transurethral bladder irrigation with 1.5% glycine solution.
- Excess antidiuretic hormone (ADH) secretion.

- Inappropriate (lung cancer, central nervous system (CNS) disorders and pulmonary sepsis).
- Appropriate (following surgery).

6. Sodium

What is the distribution of sodium in the body?

The adult body contains approximately 3000 mmol of sodium, 70% of which is free, 30% is complexed in bone. The majority of free sodium is extracellular. The normal extracellular sodium concentration is 134–145 mmol/l. The normal intracellular sodium concentration is 4–10 mmol/l.

How is sodium homoeostasis maintained?

The volume of the ECF is directly proportional to the total body sodium content. ECF volume is controlled by:

- carotid sinus baroreceptors,
- the juxtaglomerular apparatus,
- atrial natriuretic peptide.

What are you actually measuring when you measure the serum sodium?

The ratio of extracellular sodium (mmol) to extracellular water (l).

How do you assess fluid status?

Examine the patient, paying particular attention to: pulse, blood pressure (especially postural drop), jugular venous pressure (JVP), basal crackles (interstitial compartment), peripheral perfusion and oedema (interstitial compartment). Examine the charts for serial weights and fluid balance (input/output). Additional tools that may be useful include a chest radiograph (signs of pulmonary oedema), a central venous pressure (CVP) line (used dynamically) and/or a Swan–Ganz catheter.

What are the causes of hyponatraemia?

- Diarrhoea.
- Vomiting.
- Fistula.
- Burns.
- Small bowel obstruction.
- Diuretic excess.
- Addison's disease.
- Renal failure.

- Hyperosmolar diuresis.
- Water excess (usually due to intravenous (i.v.) 5% dextrose).
- Cardiac failure.
- Cirrhosis.

How do you treat hyponatraemia?

Treat the specific cause. If dehydrated, give normal saline. If not dehydrated, restrict fluids, and consider furosemide to increase water loss.

What are the complications of correcting low plasma sodium levels?

Fluid overload, secondary to excessive sodium administration which increases ECF volume and central pontine myelinosis.

What are the causes of hypernatraemia?

Hypernatraemia can be due to: water loss (diarrhoea, vomiting and burns); incorrect i.v. fluid replacement; diabetes insipidus (this may follow head injury) and osmotic diuresis.

How do you treat hypernatraemia?

Treat the cause. Give water, orally if possible. Otherwise 5% dextrose or normal saline (which is hypotonic in hypernatraemic patients).

7. Potassium

How is potassium distributed in the body?

Most potassium is intracellular. The normal serum potassium concentration is 3.5–5.0 mmol/l.

How is potassium homoeostasis maintained?

Extracellular potassium concentration is controlled primarily by the kidneys. Filtered potassium is almost completely reabsorbed in the proximal tubules.

What are the causes of hypokalaemia?

- Diuretics.
- Diarrhoea and vomiting.
- Pyloric stenosis.
- Villous adenoma of the rectum.
- Intestinal fistulae.
- Cushing's syndrome.
- Conn's syndrome.
- Purgative abuse.

How do you treat hypokalaemia?

If the serum potassium is <2.5 mmol/l, it needs urgent treatment, with cautious intravenous potassium with continuous electro-cardiography (ECG) monitoring. If the serum potassium is mild (>2.5 mmol/l), potassium may be given orally.

What are the causes of hyperkalaemia?

- Oliguric renal failure.
- Potassium sparing diuretics.
- Rhabdomyolyis.
- Burns.
- Metabolic acidosis.
- Excess potassium therapy.
- Massive blood transfusion.
- Drugs (e.g. angiotensin converting enzyme (ACE)-inhibitors and suxamethonium).

If a patient's serum potassium result came back from the laboratory as 7.1 mmol/l, what would you do?

Check that it is not an artefact, e.g. from a haemolysed sample. 10 ml of 10% calcium gluconate over 10 minutes should be given for car-dioprotection; 50 ml of 50% glucose with 20 units of insulin is then given as insulin will move potassium into the cells away from the extracellular compartment. A 5-mg salbutamol nebulizer can be tried as salbutamol activates the Na$^+$/K$^+$ ATPase, again moving extracel-luar potassium into the cells. An ECG and arterial blood gasses should be checked. The drug chart should be checked to see if there are any medications that may be causing the hyperkalemia. Calcium resonium can be given orally but further management will depend on the cause, the fluid status, renal function, and any acid/base disorder.

8. Calcium

How is calcium distributed in the body?

The adult body contains approximately 25 000 mmol of calcium, of which 99% is bound to the skeleton. The total calcium content of the ECF is 22.5 mmol, of which about 9 mmol is in the plasma. The normal serum concentration of calcium is 2.12–2.65 mmol/l. In plasma, calcium is either bound to protein (mainly albumin), complexed with citrate or phosphate, or free and physiologically active.

What are the functions of calcium in the body?

- Structural: bone and teeth.
- Neuromuscular: control of excitability, release of neurotransmitters, initiation of muscle contraction.
- Enzymes: a co-enzyme for coagulation factors.
- Signalling: an intracellular second messenger.

How is calcium homoeostasis achieved?

Calcium concentration is under the control of two hormones: parathyroid hormone (PTH) and 1,25-dihydroxycholecalciferol. A rise in PTH causes a rise in plasma calcium and a decrease in plasma phosphate. This is due to increased calcium and phosphate resorption from bone and increased calcium resorption from the kidney. PTH secretion enhances active vitamin D formation. 1,25-hydroxy-vitamin D production is stimulated by decreased calcium, decreased phosphate and PTH. It acts to increase calcium and phosphate absorption from the gut, to increase calcium and phosphate resorption in the kidney, to enhance bone turnover and inhibit PTH release.

How is serum calcium affected by pH?

In alkalosis, hydrogen ions dissociate from albumin, and calcium binding to albumin increases. There is also an increase in calcium complex formation. So, the concentration of ionised calcium falls. This is why hyperventilation causes tetany. In acidosis the opposite happens.

How is serum calcium affected by albumin?

The plasma total calcium concentration must be corrected for changes in albumin concentration.

For [albumin] <40, corrected calcium = [calcium] + 0.02 × (40 − [albumin]) mmol/l
For [albumin] >45, corrected calcium = [calcium] − 0.02 × ([albumin] − 45) mmol/l

How might hypercalcaemia present to the surgeon?

- Incidental finding.
- Non-specific musculoskeletal symptoms.
- Epigastric pain.
- Acute pancreatitis.
- Ureteric colic.
- Peptic ulcer.
- Osteoporosis.

What are the causes of hypercalcaemia?

Malignancy, with or without metastases to bone, and primary hyperparathyroidism are the commonest causes. Other causes include: renal transplantation (tertiary hyperparathyroidism), immobilisation in bone (especially Paget's disease), acromegaly and milk–alkali syndrome.

What are the features of hypocalcaemia?
- Malaise.
- Abnormal sensation and muscular excitability.
- Paraesthesia around the mouth and of the fingers.
- Hyperreflexia.
- Carpopedal spasm.
- Tetany.
- Seizures.
- Hypotension, bradycardias, dysrhythmias and congestive cardiac failure.
- Prolonged QT interval.
- Chvostek's sign.
- Trousseau's sign.

What are the causes of hypocalcaemia?
- Hypoparathyroidism (primary, secondary or most commonly post-surgical).
- Renal failure.
- Vitamin D deficiency.
- Pseudohypoparathyroidism.
- Severe magnesium deficiency.
- Acute complexing or sequestration of calcium.
- Acute pancreatitis.
- Rhabdomyolysis.

How would you manage post-parathyroidectomy hypocalcaemia?
Post-parathyroidectomy, mild hypocalcaemia normally results. This requires observation only, in the absence of symptoms. A nadir occurs at day 5 post-operatively. However, in patients who have parathyroid bone disease, a profound hypocalcaemia may occur shortly after the parathyroids are removed. This may cause a profound and severe hypocalcaemia which requires several days' treatment. If symptomatic adminster 10 ml of 10% calcium gluconate. Long-term therapy is with oral calcium and activated vitamin D (alfacacidol). The serum calcium should not exceed 2.30 mmol/l because of an increased risk of nephrolithiasis.

9. Magnesium

What is the distribution of magnesium in the body?
The adult body contains approximately 1000 mmol, half of which is in bone, one quarter in muscle and one quarter in other soft tissues.

Only 15–29 mmol is found in the ECF. The plasma concentration is 0.8–1.2 mmol/l.

What are the physiological roles of magnesium?

Magnesium acts as an essential cofactor for some 300 enzymes, involved in protein synthesis, glycolysis and transmembrane ion transport. A magnesium–adenosine triphosphate (ATP) complex is the substrate for many enzymes requiring ATP. Magnesium is important in the maintenance of the structure of ribosomes, nucleic acids and some proteins. Magnesium, by its interactions with calcium, affects the permeability of excitable membranes and their electrical properties.

When might you measure serum magnesium?

- Severe or intractable diarrhoea and/or malabsorption (e.g. short bowel syndrome and inflammatory bowel disease).
- Life-threatening alcohol withdrawal.
- Refractory cardiac dysrhythmias (especially ventricular).
- Hypocalcaemia, and/or tetany unresponsive to calcium.
- Refractory hypokalaemia.
- Neuromuscular symptoms after cisplatin or mannitol.
- Renal failure.
- During parenteral nutrition.

What are the causes of hypermagnesaemia?

Hypermagnesaemia is uncommon. Cardiac conduction is affected at concentration of 2.5–5.0 mmol/l; very high concentrations (>7.5 mmol/l) cause respiratory paralysis and cardiac arrest. Hypermagnesaemia may be seen in renal failure.

What are the causes of hypomagnesaemia?

- Malabsorption, malnutrition and fistulae.
- Alcoholism.
- Cirrhosis.
- Diuretic therapy (especially loop diuretics).
- Renal tubular disorders.
- Chronic mineralocorticoid excess.

How do you treat hypomagnesaemia?

Mild magnesium deficiency is treated with oral supplementation. In severe deficiency and with malabsorption, magnesium may be given by slow intravenous infusion.

How do you treat hypermagnesaemia?

Intravenous calcium may give short-term protection against hypermagnesaemia. In renal failure, dialysis may be necessary.

10. Functions of the Kidney

What are the functions of the kidney?
- Fluid and electrolyte balance.
- Detoxification and filtation.
- Maintenance of acid–base balance.
- Hormone production.

What hormones are produced by the kidney?
- Renin: released from the juxtaglomerular cells.
- Kallikrein: produced in the distal nephron.
- 1α-hydroxylase production: converts 25-hydroxycholecalciferol into 1,25-dihydroxycholecalciferol.
- Erythropoietin: produced in respose to anaemia.
- Prostaglandins: produced in the cortex and medulla.

What are the main buffers in the maintenance of acid–base balance?
- Proximal tubule: HCO_3^-/H_2CO_3 buffer system.
- Distal tubule: $HPO_4^{2-}/H_2PO_4^-$ buffer system.
- The phosphate buffer is the most important in normal renal function.
- NH_4^+ buffer system is the weakest buffer but allows the excretion of acid without the loss of Na^+.

Where are the sites of water reabsorbtion?
- Proximal tubule: passive transport along osmotic gradient (75% of resorbtion).
- Descending limb of loop of Henle: passive transport.
- Distal tubule: under the control of antidiuretic hormone (ADH).
- Collecting ducts: under the control of ADH.

How is the osmolality of urine controlled?
The concentration of urine is under the control of ADH on the collecting duct. ADH increases permeability and results in increased water resorbtion. Osmolality varies between 50 and 1200 mosmol/l.

11. Glomerulus

Can you describe the glomerulus?
The glomerulus is formed by a group of capillaries, supplied by an afferent arteriole, invaginating into the Bowman's capsule and drained by an efferent arteriole.

What is the function of the glomerular membrane?

The glomerular membrane allows passage of neutral substances up to 4nm in diameter into the Bowman's capsule and excludes substances with a diameter of over 8nm, though the charge of the substance also affects its passage across the membrane. (The endothelium of the glomerulus is fenestrated and contains pores 70–90nm wide and the glomerular epithelium contains filtration slits 25nm.)

How is the glomerular filtration rate (GFR) measured?

The GFR can be measured by measuring the extraction and plasma level of a substance that is freely filtered through the glomeruli and is neither secreted nor reabsorbed by the renal tubules. The total amount of plasma filtered through the glomeruli is 170–180l/day. GFR is approximately 125ml/minute.

What substances can be used to measure GFR?

Inulin can be used to measure GFR (inulin is a fructose polymer).

What are the factors that increase GFR?

- Increased renal blood flow.
- Increased capillary hydrostatic pressure.
- Increased afferent arteriolar pressure.
- Decreased efferent arteriolar pressure.
- Increased glomerular permeability.
- Hypoproteinemia.

What factors decrease GFR?

The opposite of any of the factors listed in the question above, and:

- Decrease systemic blood pressure (<90mmHg).
- Ureteric obstruction.
- Oedema of the kidney.
- Dehydration.
- Decrease in effective filtration surface area.

12. Loop of Henle

What is the function of the loop of Henle?

- Descending limb: water, Na^+ and Cl^- are reabsorbed.
- Ascending limb: impermeable to water but Na^+ and Cl^- are reabsorbed.
- Formation of countercurrent multipliers.

What are the different types of loop of Henle?

Long (juxtamedullary nephrons) and short (cortical nephrons) loops.
In man 15% of nephrons have long loops.

Which are important in the formation of a countercurrent multiplier?

The long loops, the longer the loop the greater the osmolality at its tip.

What is the advantage of this countercurrent mulitplier?

A high osmotic gradient is formed across the kidney with the cortex
being isotonic and the medulla hypotonic. This allows a very dilute
urine to be produced in the distal tubule.

GASTROINTESTINAL PHYSIOLOGY

13. Gastric Secretions

What volume of gastric secretions are produced each day by a healthy adult?
Approximately 2500 ml.

What are the contents of gastric secretions?
- Hydrochloric acid.
- Papsin.
- Gastric lipase.
- Intrinsic factor.
- Mucus.
- Water.
- Ions (e.g. Na^+, K^+, Mg^{2+}, HPO_4^{2-}, SO_4^{2-}).

What is the function of hydrochloric acid?
- Activate pepsinogen to pepsin.
- Convert ferric acid to ferrous form.
- Acid environment aids the absorption of calcium.
- Killing of ingested bacteria.

Which cells secrete pepsin?
The chief cells secrete it as an inactive precursor pepsinogen.

What is the function of pepsin?
Breaks down food proteins to peptides and polypeptides.

Which cells secrete intrinsic factor?
The parietal cells.

What is the function of intrinsic factor?
Binds to vitamin B_{12} so that it can be absorbed by the ileal mucosal epithelial cells.

How is acid secretion regulated?
There three phases to acid secretion: cephalic, gastric and intestinal phases.

- Cephalic phase: initiated by the site, smell taste or thought of food. Vagally mediated, acetylcholine directly stimulates the production of acid and indirectly causes acid secretion by stimulating secretion of gastrin (from G cells) and histamine (enterochromaphin-like cells).

- Gastric phase: the mechanical effect of food in the stomach, distension of the body, antrum and pyloric area leads to the release of gastrin and also causes vagal stimulation leading to stimulation of parietal cells. Protein digestion products, calciun ions, caffeine, alcohol and amino acids in the antrum stimulate gastric secretions.
- Intestinal phase: duodenal distension, presence of peptides and amino acids stimulates gastric secretion mainly by G cells in the duodenum. Acid in the duodenum leads to the release of secretin, fatty acids in the duodenum causes the release of cholecystokinin (CCK) and gastric inhibitory peptide all of which inhibit gastric secretion.

14. Bile

How much bile is produced a day?
Bile is produced 500–1500 ml/day and is stored in the gall bladder between meals.

What is the function of bile?
- Bile salts are required for lipid digestion.
- HCO_3^- aids neutralisation of gastric acid as it enters the duodenum.
- Excretory route for bile pigment, cholesterol, steroids and fat-soluble drugs. .

How do bile salts function?
Hepatocytes form primary bile salts (steroid molecules) from cholesterol. Primary bile salts are dehydroxylated by intestinal bacteria to secondary bile salts. Bile salts are detergents (containing a fat and a water-soluble end), in aqueous solutions bile salts form micelles (hydrophobic ends in the centre and the hydrophilic ends on the surface) this enables them to solubalise and assist the absorption of lipids.

Where are bile salts absorbed?
Eighty per cent of bile salts are absorbed actively in the distal ileum and pass back to the liver via the portal circulation. The remaining bile salts enter the colon where they are converted to secondary bile salts (deoxycholate-soluble and lithocholate-insoluble) and the soluble deoxycholate is absorbed. The bile salts that are not absorbed (mainly lithocholate) are excreted in the faeces.

Ninety per cent of bile salts secreted are reabsorbed. Bile salts are recycled up to eight times a day.

What are bile pigments and how are they excreted?

Degradation of the haem group of haemoglobin leads to the formation of biliverdin. This is then reduced to unconjugated bilirubin and is taken to liver attached to albumin. Unconjugated bilirubin is conjugated with glucuronic acid in the liver. This is now water-soluble and is excreted in bile. Intestinal bacteria reduce the conjugated bilirubin to urobilinogen (absorbed and returns to the liver and is excreted into the bile) and stercobilinogen (excreted in faeces).

15. Duodenum

What are the functions of the duodenum?
- Control of gastric contents.
- Stimulation of gastric acid.
- Reduction in gastric acid output.
- Pancreatic secretion stimulation.
- Stimulates bile formation.
- Stimulation of gall bladder contraction.
- Absorption of carbohydrates, amino acids, fatty acids, calcium and some vitamin.

How is gastric acid output affected by the duodenum?
Gastrin released by the duodenal G cells stimulates gastric acid secretion.

Secretin and gastric inhibitory peptide secreted by duodenal S and M cells respectively reduce the secretion of gastrin in the stomach and therefore reduce gastric acid secretion.

How does the duodenum control gastric acid?
The mucosa of the duodenum is more resistant to the gastric acid. The duodenum is where neutralisation of gastric acid occurs.

How does neutralisation of gastric acid occur?
Pancreatic secretions containing HCO_3^- are stimulated by secretin and CCK released from the duodenum. CCK also stimulates gall bladder contraction and bile formation. HCO_3^- is also secreted from the glands of Brunner in the submucosa.

What are the effects of duodenectomy?
- Acid contents reaching the jejunum can cause ulceration.
- Incomplete neutralisation leading to decreased absorption of iron, calcium and phosphate.
- Loss of control of gastric emptying can lead to dumping syndrome.
- Loss of pancreatic and biliary stimulation leads decreased fat absorption.

What is dumping syndrome?
Dumping syndrome can be caused by excessive volumes of food entering the small intestine to fast. This leads to large volumes of extracellular fluid into the lumen of the intestine and uncontrolled carbohydrate absorption leading to rapid changes in serum glucose. Symptoms include faintness, sweating, abdominal pain and tachycardia.

16. Pancreas

How much pancreatic fluid is secreted each day?
Pancreatic fluid is secreted 1500 ml/day.

What do pancreatic secretions contain?
Water, electrolytes (Cations: Na^+, K^+, Ca^{2+} and Mg^{2+}. Anions: HCO_3^-, Cl^-, SO_4^{2-}, HPO_4^{2-}. pH around 8) and enzymes.

Can you name the important pancreatic enzymes?
- Trypsinogen: breaks down proteins to polypeptides and peptides, converted to the active form trypsin by enterokinase in the duodenum, trypsin also actives tripsinogen.
- Pancreatic amylase: breaks down starch and glycogen.
- Pancreatic lipase: breaks down triglycerides to monoglycerides and fatty acids.

How are pancreatic secretions regulated?
Pancreatic secretions are controlled by a number of hormonal and neuronal mechanisms:

- Secretin: produced by endocrine cells in the duodenum and jejunum, it stimulates the secretion of an alkaline fluid high in HCO_3^- and low in enzymes.
- CCK: produced by endocrine cells in the duodenum and jejunum, it acts on acinar cells leading to the release zymogen granules, producing pancreatic secretions high in enzyme content.

- Acetylcholine: acts on acinar cells.
- Vagal stimulation: causes release of pancreatic secretions high in enzymes content.
- Somatostatin: released from pancreatic islet D cells, inhibits pancreatic secretions.

What are the endocrine functions of the pancreas?

The following hormones are secreted by the islets of Langerhans:

- Insulin: produced by the β cells, it facilitating glucose uptake to muscle, glycogen and fat synthesis in the liver. It also inhibits glycogen breakdown.
- Glucagon: produced by the α cells, it stimulates glycogenolysis and gluconeogenesis in the liver.
- Somatostatin: released from pancreatic islet D cells, it inhibits insulin and glucagon release. It also inhibits pancreatic and gastric secretions.
- Pancreatic polypeptide: has a role in gastrointestinal function.

What would the effects of subtotal or total pancreotectomy be?

Removal of all, or almost all, of the pancreas will lead to a varying degree of malabsorption of fat. This will result in failure to absorb fat-soluble vitamins such as A, D, E and K, and, if not supplemented, may result in vitamin deficiency. Protein malnutrition may ensue and without proper glucose control patients may develop glucose intolerance and diabetes.

17. Liver

What are the functions of the liver?

- Production and secretion of bile.
- Synthesis of plasma proteins.
- Metabolism of proteins, fats, carbohydrates and vitamins.
- Storage of glycogen, iron, copper and vitamins (A, D, E, K and B_{12}).
- Detoxification of toxins, steroids and hormones.
- Reticulo-endothelial function.
- Haeopoiesis in the foetus.

What plasma proteins are synthesised by the liver?

- Acute phase proteins.
- Albumin.
- Proteins that transport steroids.

- Proteins that transport hormones.
- Clotting factors V, VII, IX and X.

How are substances inactivated and excreted by the liver?

The liver reduces the toxicity and biological activity of substances and increases their water-solubility. The cytochrome P450 system is involved in increasing water-solubility. The formation of glucoronides of a variety of substances including bilirubin, steroids and some drugs is catalyzed by the glucuronyl transferase system.

What substances affect the cytochrome P450 system?

- Increase activity is caused by: barbituates, phenytoin and rifampicin.
- Decrease activity is caused by: erythromycin, ketoconazole and cimetidine.

What cells carry out the reticuloendothelial function in the liver?

Kupffer cells remove bacteria, toxins and abnormal erythrocytes.

18. Small Bowel

What substances are absorbed or digested by the small intestines?

- Water and electrolytes.
- Carbohydrates.
- Protein.
- Fat.
- Iron.
- Folate.
- Calcium.
- Vitamin B_{12}.

How is vitamin B_{12} absorbed?

Vitamin B_{12} is found in animal food sources. In the stomach it combines with intrinsic factor produced by the parietal cells. This complex is then absorbed in the terminal ileum.

What factors reduce absorption of intrinsic factors?

- Lack of intrinsic factor (pernicious anaemia and gastric resection).
- Loss of terminal ileum (resection and Crohn's disease).
- Blind loop syndrome.

What are the causes of malabsorption?

- Abnormal digestion in the intestinal lumen.
- Pyloroplasty: dumping syndrome (inadequate mixing of food with pancreatic secretions and bile).
- Small bowel resection: reduced absorptive area.
- Chronic pancreatitis.
- Cystic fibrosis.
- Blockage of bile duct (stone and carcinoma).
- Excess gastric secretion: leading to inadequate lipolysis.
- Blind loop syndrome: causing bacterial overgrowth decreasing conjugated bile salts.
- Celiac disease.
- Disaccharide deficiency.
- Abnormal fat transport in the lymphatics.

How much small bowel is necessary for survival?

Only 80 cm is required.

What are the consequences of small bowel resection?

After loss of most of the jejunum fat, protein and carbohydrate absorption is reduced due to the loss of absorptive area. This leads to diarrhoea with loss of water and electrolytes. The ileum over several weeks adjusts taking over most of the functions of the jejunum after resection. When over 1 m of terminal ileum is resected bile salts and vitamin B_{12} absorption is reduced and the jejunum is not able to compensate. Stores of vitamin B_{12} last over 3 years, the bile salt pool however declines, this leads to increased gallstone formation, steatorrhoea and decreased absorption of fat-soluble vitamin (A, D, E and K).

19. Large Bowel

What are the main functions of the large intestine?

- Absorption.
- Secretion.
- Motility.
- Storage.

What does the large bowel absorb?

Water: 1–2 l enter the colon a day and only 100–200 ml are excreted.

- Electrolytes: Na^+ is actively absorbed.
- Amino acids.
- Fatty acids.
- Vitamin K and B complex vitamins.

What is secreted from the large bowel?
- Electrolytes: K^+ and HCO_3^- are secreted.
- Mucus: secreted by the goblet cells.

What is stored in the colon?
Faeces are stored mainly in the transverse colon until defection occurs. Gas mainly consisting of nitrogen, it also contains oxygen, carbon dioxide, methane (only 1% of the population) and hydrogen sulphide.

What are the consequences of diarrhoea?
In the acute situation absorption of Na^+ and water and reduced secretion of K^+ and HCO_3^- is reduced. This leads to dehydration and metabolic acidosis. In chronic diarrhoea aldosterone leads to increase K^+ loss from the kidneys and large bowel, causing hypokalaemia and a metabolic alkalosis.

What are the causes of diarrhoea?
- Reduced absorptive capacity (bowel resection and colitis).
- Malabsorption.
- Excess bile.
- Increased peristalsis.
- Infection.
- Tumours (carcinoid).
- Drugs (laxatives and antibiotics).

ENDOCRINE PHYSIOLOGY

20. Thyroid Gland

Briefly describe the synthesis of tri-iodothyronine (T3) and thyroxine (T4).

Iodide in the blood is taken up by the iodide pump present in thyroid follicular epithelial cells. The iodide is oxidised by thyroidal peroxidase and is transported within the cell. Here, the newly formed iodine is linked to tyrosine residues in the protein thyroglobulin. It is then secreted into the colloid at the centre of each follicle (a thyroid follicle is colloid surrounded by thyroid follicular cells). At the junction of the follicular cells and the lumen further action by peroxidase converts the tyrosine residues to mono-iodotyrosine (MIT) and di-iodotyrosine (DIT). MIT then couples with DIT to form T3 and DIT couples with DIT to form T4. Thyro-globulin is stored within the colloid until the gland is stimulated to secrete thyroid hormone. The stores typically last for 2 months. When thyroid hormones are required, thyroglobulin is redirected into the follicular cell by pinocytosis. Proteases act on thyroglobulin to produce T3 and T4, which are then released into the circulation. Thyroid-stimulating hormone (TSH) stimulates each step in the synthesis of T3 and T4. The remaining MIT and DIT is deiodinated by thyroid deiodinase. The I_2 released is recycled to synthesise more thyroid hormones.

How are T3 and T4 transported in the bloodstream?

In the bloodstream T3 and T4 are bound predominantly to thyroxine-binding globulin (TBG) but also to albumin and thyroid-binding pre-albumin. More T4 is produced than T3 and in the peripheral tissues T4 is converted to T3 by 5′-iodinase.

Which is more biologically active, T3 or T4?

T3 is at least four times as potent as T4. However, T3 has a much shorter half-life – approximately 1 day compared with 1 week for T4.

How is thyroid hormone secretion controlled?

TSH has a direct positive effect on thyroid hormone production. TSH is secreted from the anterior pituitary and is itself regulated by thyroid releasing hormone (TRH) secreted by the hypothalamus. TRH is produced in response to low circulating thyroid hormone concentration and a fall in external temperature. The hypothalamus–pituitary–thyroid axis works by negative feedback, i.e. thyroid hormone production inhibits TRH secretion from the hypothalamus and TSH secretion from the anterior pituitary. The thyroid gland itself shows some ability to autoregulate depending on the iodine supply. High iodine circulating levels are inhibitory to thyroid hormone production. Deficiency states in endemic regions are associated with goitre as the glands infrastructure swells in an attempt to produce thyroid hormones.

What are the effects of thyroid hormones in the body?

Thyroid hormones are steroid hormones and work by increasing DNA transcription in cells with a resultant increase in new mRNA. The new mRNA is translated into the production of new specific proteins that have physiological actions. These effects are widespread in the human body and can be summarised as follows:

- Central nervous system (CNS) maturation: this is totally dependent on thyroid hormone production in the perinatal period. Lack of hormone or deficiency can result in mental retardation and cretinism and as a result hypothyroidism is screened for in the neonatal period.
- Growth and skeletal maturation: thyroid and growth hormones act synergistically to promote bone formation and maturation.
- Regulation of basal metabolic rate (BMR) and temperature regulation: thyroid hormones cause increased oxygen consumption by mitochondria with a subsequent increase in adenosine triphosphate (ATP) formation in most organs of the body (not brain, spleen or gonads). This causes an increase in heat production indirectly and therefore explains why thyrotoxic patients complain of heat intolerance. Thyroid hormones influence BMR directly i.e. patients with hypothyroidism have a low BMR and vice versa.
- Metabolic effects: there is a net increase in protein breakdown and hence thyroid hormones are catabolic. There is an increase in fat mobilisation and degradation. Glucose absorption is promoted from the gastrointestinal tract and there is an increase in glycogenolysis and gluconeogenesis.
- Sympathomimetic: many effects of thyroid hormone are analogous to β adrenergic stimulation. This explains how thyrotoxic patients can get some symptomatic relief with β blockers.
- Other effects: thyroid hormones cause an increase in stroke volume and heart rate. Since these two parameters have an effect on cardiac output, this too increases. This in combination with increased ventilation, another effect of thyroid hormones, promotes increased oxygen delivery to tissues. Thyroid hormones also play a role in regulation of gut motility and skin/hair development.

What is the pathophysiology of Graves' disease?

Graves disease is an autoimmune condition in which high circulating levels of thyroid-stimulating immunoglobulins or long acting thyroid stimulators (LATS) are present. These antibodies are directed at the TSH receptor and are stimulatory. As a result thyroid hormone levels in these patients are raised. They present with generalised hyperthyroid symptoms, symptoms specific to Graves (exopthalmos, acropachy and pretibial myxoedema) or a combination of both. TSH levels are low due to the negative feedback mechanism.

21. Parathyroid Glands

What actions does parathyroid hormone (PTH) have?

PTH is secreted in response to a reduced sereum calcium. It promotes resorption of bone, reabsorption of calcium in the distal convuluted tubule of the kidney and increases production of 1,25-dihydroxycholecalciferol. All these processes act to increase the serum calcium. Increased 1,25-dihydroxycholecalciferol production in the kidney has a direct effect on increasing intestinal absorption of calcium. The bone resorption effect promotes an increase in both phosphate and calcium in the extracelleular fluid. Normally 40% of calcium is bound to plasma proteins and the other 60% is filtered by the kidney. The filtered load is either bound to anions or is free ionised calcium. PTH promotes phosphate excretion in the proximal convuluted tubule and since phosphate complexes calcium, this action of PTH helps to increase free uncomplexed calcium, which is the biologically active form.

What is the active form of vitamin D and describe its synthesis and its effects?

Vitamin D is ingested in our diet as cholecalciferol. 7-dehydrocholesterol in our skin, by the action of ultraviolet light, also contributes to the production of cholecalciferol. Cholecalciferol is inactive but when it reaches the liver it is converted to 25-hydroxycholecalciferol, another inactive metabolite, by the action of 25α-hydroxylase. This in turn is converted to 1,25-dihydroxycholecalciferol (active form) and 24,25-dihydroxycholecalciferol (inactive form) in the kidney by the action of 1α-hydroxylase enzyme. 1α-hydroxylase activity is increased by a reduced serum calcium or phosphate or by a raised PTH level. 1,25-dihydroxycholecalciferol then promotes calcium and phosphate reabsorption in the kidney and intestine and promotes bone resorption.

What are the causes of primary hyperparathyroidism?
- Parathyroid adenoma (85%).
- Parathyroid hyperplasia (14%).
- Parathyroid carcinoma (1%).

What is the net biochemical changes in primary hyperparathyroidism?
Primary hyperparathyroidism leads to a raised serum calcium, PTH level and a decresed serum phosphate.

What are the signs and symptoms of primary hyperparathyroidism?
Although some patients may be asymptomatic, many will show the effetcs of hypercalcaemia:

- Weakness, fatigue, nausea and vomiting.
- Polyuria, polydypsia and dehydration.
- Renal calculi.
- Abdominal pain, peptic ulcer disease, pancreatitis and constipation.
- Cardiac dysrhythmias.
- Renal impairment.
- Corneal and vascular deposits.
- Psychiatric illness (depression).
- Bony conditions: skeletal pain, fractures, subperosteal erosions especially of phalanges and cystic lesions.

How can primary hyperparathyroidism be treated?
Treatment can involve surgical exploration with removal of the offending gland in cases of adenoma or carcinoma. With hyperplastic glands, three and a half glands out of the four are removed in order for symptomatic control. In asymptomatic disease the debate still continues whether surgery should be undertaken as long-term sequelae are still possible.

How does renal failure cause secondary hyperparathyroidism and what serum biochemical will ensue?
In renal failure glomerular filtration is reduced and phosphate excretion is hampered. As a result more phosphate is available to bing to calcium and thus the free or ionised calcium pool is reduced and patients tend to become hypocalcaemic. There is a reduction in active vitamin D formation which also prevents intestinal absorption of

calcium, confounding the problem. The body's response to this is to try and increase serum calcium. It achieves this by increasing parathyroid hormone and eventually this leads to secondary hyperparathyroidism (i.e. an increase in PTH in response to low serum calcium). The increased bone resorption in combination with reduced intestinal absorption eventually leads to osteomalacia and produces the apt named renal ostedystrophy seen in these patients. The biochemical will include a raised parathyroid hormone level and phosphate level with a decreased serum calcium level.

What are the causes of hypoparathyroisdism and what biochemical changes would occur in primary disease?

- Neck surgery (e.g. thyroid surgery).
- Congenital conditions (e.g. Albrights hereditary osteodystrophy).
- Primary hypoparathyroidism causes a low PTH, with a low serum calcium and a raised serum phosphate.

22. Adrenal Glands

What important hormones are secreted from the different layers of the adrenal gland?

The adrenal cortex has three distinct zones: zona glomerulosa – secretes aldosterone, zona fasiculata – secretes glucocorticoids (e.g. cortisol) and the zona reticularis – secretes sex hormones (e.g. testosterone and oestrogen). The adrenal medulla secretes catecholamines such as adrenaline and noradrenaline.

What are the actions of cortisol?

Cortisol is a catabolic hormone and is essential in the body's response to stress. Its actions are as follows:

- Anti-inflammatory: induces synthesis of lipocortin which acts on the arachodonic metabolite pathway inhibiting the enzyme phospholipase A2. This enzymes liberates arachodonic acid from free phospholipids and goes on to produce the mediators of pain and inflammation (leucotrienes, prostaglandins and thromboxanes). In addition, it inhibits proliferation of T lymphocytes, prevents the production of interleukin-2 and prevents mast cells and platelets secreting histamine and serotonin respectively.
- Promotes protein catabolism and lipolysis: this makes more amino acids and glycerol are available in the liver for gluconeogenesis.

- Reduction in insulin sensitivity.
- Enhances the effect of catecholamine on the peripheral vasculature: noradrenaline causes vasoconstriction in the peripheral vasculature and this effect is potentiated by cortisol. In Addison's disease, where there is a distinct lack of cortisol, the peripheral effect of noradrenaline is diminished and patients therefore tend to develop postural hypotension.

How is glucocorticoid secretion regulated?

Cortisol levels vary during a normal day, being highest in the morning. Cortisol secretion is dependent on stimulation of the adrenal cortex by adrenocorticotrophic hormone (ACTH). ACTH in turn is secreted from the anterior pituitary in response to corticotrophin releasing hormone which is secreted from the hypothalamus. The system like other hypo-thalomo-pituitary-end organ axis is governed by negative feedback such that raised cortisol levels will cause a suppression I the amount of corticotrophin releasing hormone (CRH) and ACTH released from the hypothalamus and anterior pituitary respectively.

What are the actions of aldosterone?

- Increases Na^+ reabsorption in the distal convuluted tubule and collecting system of the kidney.
- Incresaes potassium secretion in the distal convuluted tubulae and collecting system of the kidney.
- Promotes secretion of H^+ ions (acid) from the kidney.

How does aldosterone contribute to the homoeostasis of the extracellular fluid compartment in hypovolaemic states?

A reduction in tissue perfusion of the kidneys secondary to a reduc-tion in blood volume stimulates the renin–angiotensin system. As a result a surge in renin production occurs which causes angiotensinogen to be converted to angiotensin I. This is then converted to angiotensin II by the action of angiotensin converting enzyme. Angiotensin II is a potent vasoconstrictor (helping to maintain mean arterial pressure) and also acts on the zona glomerulosa of the adrenal cortex to stimu-late secretion of aldosterone. Aldosterone promotes Na^+ reabsorption in the kidney. Along with this shift comes a shift in water thereby restoring the extracellular fluid volume towards normal.

What is Addison's disease?

Addison's disease or primary adrenocortical insufficiency is usually due to autoimmune destruction of the adrenal cortex. Other causes include tuberculosis, adrenal adenoma/carcinoma and sudden with-drawal of steroids. As a result the adrenal gland is unable to produce the mineralocorticoid, aldosterone; glucocorticoids such as cortisol or sex hormones. The symptoms therefore expressed are related to their relevant deficiencies. Treatment is with mineralocorticoid and gluco-corticoid replacement. Despite this patients tend to develop adrenal crises when the body undergoes further stresses such as surgery, infection and immunosuppression.

What are the clinical features of Addison's disease?

- General: nausea, vomiting, weight loss, anorexia, malaise and weakness.
- ACTH related: in producing higher circulating level of ACTH, melanocyte-stimulating hormone (MSH) levels are also increased leading to hyperpigmentation which tends to manifest in the peri-oral region.
- Aldosterone related: postural hypotension (secondary to a reduction in extracellular fluid volume), hyperkalaemia, metabolic acidosis (aldosterone promotes acid secretion and therefore conversely leads to acidosis in aldosterone deficient states).
- Hyponatraemia.
- Cortisol related: hypoglycaemia, loss of cortisol induced peripheral vasoconstrictor effect with noradrenaline (contributing to postural hypotension).
- Sex hormone related: reduced pubic and axillary hair in women.

23. Hydraulic Filter

What is the principle function of the arterial system?
To distribute blood to the capillary beds throughout the body ensuring tissue perfusion.

What do you understand by the term "hydraulic filtering" in relation to the arterial system?
Hydraulic filtering is a term that relates to the conversion of the intermittent, pulsatile outflow of blood from the heart to a steady flow through the capillaries.

What advantage is there from hydraulic filtering in the arterial system?
Hydraulic filtering reduces the amount of work required to perfuse tissues.

What features of the arterial system produce hydraulic filtering?
There are two features: the compliance of the great vessels and regulation of flow by high resistance arterioles.

Do you know of any classic analogies to hydraulic filtering?
Hydraulic filtering has classically been compared to the Windkessel of a steam engine which is a compressible air trap which converts the intermittent flow of water to a steady outflow.

24. Arterial Pressure

What is blood pressure?
Blood pressure is the pressure developed by blood flow and can be expressed in either of two ways: as a ratio of systolic over diastolic pressure (SBP/DBP) or as mean arterial pressure (MAP).

What factors determine arterial blood pressure?
In broad terms, the factors determining arterial pressure can be divided into physical factors (blood volume and compliance) and physiological factors (cardiac output (CO), heart rate, stroke volume (SV), vascular resistance, etc.).

How can CO and systemic vascular resistance (SVR) affect blood pressure?

Essentially, in any given artery the MAP will be proportional to the volume of blood. CO and SVR can be understood to affect MAP by how they might alter the volume of blood. CO is the inflow of blood to the artery (CO = inflow) and SVR is inversely proportional to the outflow of blood from the artery (SVR = 1/outflow). An increase in either CO or SVR will, therefore, increase blood volume and, therefore, MAP. Or in other words, MAP = CO × SVR.

What is pulse pressure (PP)?

PP is the difference between SBP and DBP (PP = SBP − DBP).

What factors affect PP and why they are important?

Two main factors determine PP: SV and compliance. As pressure is proportional to the volume of the blood in the artery an increase in SV will produce a proportionate increase in PP. Provided compliance is normal, therefore, PP can give information about SV (therefore PP is reduced in patients who have suffered severe haemorrhage for example). A reduction in compliance will increase PP for a given SV. This is significant in patients with atherosclerosis as a greater workload is placed on the left ventricle. A similar situation arises in hypertensive patients as compliance is reduced at higher pressures.

25. Haemodynamics

How are pressure and flow related in blood vessels?

Poiseuille's law determines the flow of fluids through cylindrical tubes. It is applicable to Newtonian fluids with steady laminar flow. Poiseuille's law states:

$$\text{Flow} = \Delta P \pi r^4 / 8 \Gamma l$$

where P = Pressure.
r = Radius of vessel.
l = Length of vessel.
Γ = Viscosity of fluid.

Are there any other laws relating to blood flow that can be applied?

Yes, ohms law can be applied: $\Delta P = \text{Flow} \times \text{SVR}$. If this law is applied to the systemic circulation then BP = CO × SVR.

Where is the greatest vascular resistance in the systemic circulation?

The small arteries and arterioles. SVR is regulated mainly by the arterioles.

What is the significance of a parallel arrangement of capillary beds?

A parallel arrangement of capillary beds allows for oxygenated blood to perfuse all beds and there can be independent of regulation of blood flow to each individual bed. Also, the total SVR is determined by the collective the resistance in all capillary beds in the following way: $1/SVR = 1/R_1 + 1/R_2 = 1/R_3$ etc. ($R_{1,2,3}$ are the resistances in the respective capillary beds).

What is meant to be velocity and flow in a blood vessel and how are these two properties related?

Velocity refers the speed of individual components of blood (m/second) whereas flow refers to the quantity of blood passing through the vessel per unit time. They are related in the following way: Flow = velocity × cross-sectional area.

How does arterial stenosis affect blood flow and velocity?

Stenosis causes increased resistance to flow and produces a pressure drop across the stenosed area (pressure proximal to stenosis >pressure distal to stenosis). Assuming that flow remains constant, velocity will increase through the area of stenosis. As velocity increases there is a risk that smooth lamina flow will change to turbulent flow. Reynold's number (N_R is used to estimate the likelihood of turbulent flow (when $N_R > 3000$ flow will be turbulent).

What is meant by critical stenosis and when does it occur?

Arterial stenosis is said to be critical when the flow rate reduces through the area of stenosis. This point usually occurs when there is around 70% stenosis.

26. Principles of Vascular Control

What factors control blood flow though a capillary bed?

These factors can be classified into metabolic, hormonal, neural and physical factors. Metebolic factors include lactate, H^+, and CO_2.

Hormonal factors include cortisol and adrenaline. Neural factors include sympathetic and parasympathetic outflow, baroreceptors and chemoreceptors. Physical factors include CO and comliance. All these factors can modulate blood flow through a capillary bed either directly, indirectly or both.

Can you name some circulating factors that can cause vasodilatation and some that cause vasoconstriction?

- Vasodilatation: somatostatin, histamine and bradykinin.
- Vasoconstriction: angiotension II and adrenaline.

Can you do the same for endothelial-derived factors?

- Vasodilatation: nitric oxide; prostaglandin I_2 (PGI_2).
- Vasoconstriction: endothelin and thromboxane.

Can you do the same for neurotransmitters?

- Vasodilatation: adenosine triphosphate (ATP), vasoactive intestinal peptide (VIP) and substance P.
- Vasoconstriction: noradrenaline.

Can you do the same for metabolic factors?

- Vasodilatation: K^+ and CO_2.
- Vasoconstriction: Ca^{2+}.

Are there any important key elements in the control of vascular smooth muscle tone?

There is an intimate relationship with the endothelial lining with a number of signals from the circulation being transmitted to VSM through an effect on the endothelium. The contractile elements in VSM are more disorganised than those in striated muscle and this may facilitate longer periods of contraction in VSM. There are a variety of voltage- and receptor-operated channels (VOC's and ROC's, respectively) which allow an influx of Ca^{2+} into VSM cells. The types of VOC's and ROC's in different capillary beds will all different responses to the same stimulus.

27. Cardiac Cell Physiology

Which three ions are associated with the cardiac action potential?

Na^+, K^+ and Ca^{2+}.

What are the intracellular and extracellular concentration of each of these?

Ions	Extracellular concentration (mM)	Intracellular concentration (mM)
K^+	4	135
Na^+	145	10
Ca^{2+}	2	10^{-4}

What is the resting potential of a cardiac cell and how do you account for this?

Approximately $-80\,mV$.

The cell membrane is permeable to K^+ but less permeable to the anions (e.g. proteins) within the cells. In the resting state K^+ ions leave the cell and anions are left behind, making the interior of the cell electronegative.

Can you describe the movement of these ions across the cardiac cell membrane during depolarisation?

Triggering of the action potential by the pacemaker cells results in a brief increase in cell membrane permeability to Na^+ ions. There is rapid influx of Na^+ ions making the transmembrane potential positive. K^+ then diffuses out of the cell to restore negative transmembrane potential (repolarisation). Restoration of membrane potential is delayed by influx of Ca^{2+} ions (plateau phase of action potential). This means that there is an obligatory period during which the cell cannot be depolarised – this prevents tetany.

What are the effects of hyperkalaemia on the heart?

A large increase in extracellular K^+ results in loss of cell excitation, decreased rate of conduction and slowing of the heart with dysrythmias.

28. Cardiac Cycle

What is the cardiac cycle?

The cardiac cycle relates events within the heart to simple body-surface measurements. The opening and closing of the heart valves, and pressure changes within the chambers of the heart (and aorta and jugular vein) are drawn in relation to the timing of heart sounds and changes on an electrocardiography (ECG) trace.

How long is the cardiac cycle in seconds?
It is 0.4 seconds.

What cardiac event does the p wave on an ECG relate to?
Atrial depolarisation.

What cardiac event does the QRS complex on an ECG relate to?
Ventricular depolarisation.

With regard to the left ventricle, what are the phases of the cardiac cycle?
Left ventricular contraction and relaxation. Left ventricular contraction can be further divided into phases of isovolumetric contraction, rapid ejection and slow ejection. Left ventricular relaxation can be further subdivided into phases of reduced ejection, isovolumetric relaxation, rapid filling and slow filling.

What is the difference between cardiological and physiological left ventricular systole?
Cardiological left ventricular systole is defined as the period between closure of the mitral and aortic valve. Physiological left ventricular systole is defined as isovolumetric contraction to the end of the rapid ejection phase.

29. Control of Cardiac Output (CO)

What is the CO of a normal 70 kg man at rest?
The CO is 5 l/minute.

What formula is typically used to represent this value?
$Q = HR \times SV$

where Q = CO (l/minute).
         HR = Heart rate (beats/minute).
         SV = Stroke volume (l).

What is Starling's law?

The force of contraction of the heart is proportional to the length of its muscle fibres, i.e. increasing venous return to the heart results in increase stretch of the muscle fibres and in turn a greater force of contraction, therefore increasing SV. There is, however, an optimum fibre length and excessive stretch will depress pumping capacity.

What are the effects of sympathetic stimulation on CO?

Increased myocardial contractility and increased heart rate and, therefore, a rise in CO.

30. Shock and Inotropes

Can you define shock?

This refers to insufficient organ perfusion and inadequate oxygen delivery to tissues.

How many different types of shock do you know?

Haemorrhagic, cardiogenic, spinal, anaphylactic and septic shock.

Can you describe the mechanisms involved in septic shock?

This is caused by endotoxins released by gram-negative organisms. These impair the ability of cells to utilise oxygen and also cause vasodilatation. In this situation shock can occur despite adequate or even high oxygen delivery. The endotoxin acts on capillaries to render them "leaky" and this together with vasodilatation can result in profound hypovolaemia. Endotoxins are also negatively inotropic.

What are the signs that may distinguish septic from haemorrhagic shock?

The septic patient is often pyrexial, with warm periphery and may have a high CO. In haemorrhagic shock the patient is cold and clammy, peripherally shut down and is likely to have a low CO.

Which inotrope is commonly used to treat septic shock?

Noradrenaline. This agent predominantly acts on α_1 receptors to cause vasoconstriction and raise total peripheral resistance thus increasing systolic and diastolic blood pressure (SBP and DBP).

31. Blood Pressure Regulation

Can you define mean arterial pressure using a simple equation?

$$MAP = CO \times TPR$$

where   CO = Cardiac output (l/minute).

TPR = Total peripheral resistance (dyne seconds/cm^5).

Which sites account for the majority of resistance in the circulation?

The capillaries and arterioles. The former have a narrow calibre, a large surface area and are numerous. The latter are lined with smooth muscle which can contract, narrowing the vessel and increasing resistance.

Where are the baroreceptors that monitor blood pressure located?

In the carotid sinus and the aortic arch.

How do these receptors respond to a fall in blood pressure?

These stretch receptors respond to a fall in pressure by reducing afferent signals carried via the IX and X cranial nerves to the cardiac and vasomotor centres in the medulla. This results in increased sympathetic activity via the autonomic system and reduced vagal tone. The consequence of this is vasoconstriction, increased heart rate and stroke volume. This raises both total peripheral resistance and CO, restoring blood pressure.

How does transection of the cord at the level of T6 lead to "spinal shock"?

Loss of sympathetic tone results in profound vasodilatation and a fall in total peripheral resistance. In addition, unimpeded vagal drive causes bradycardia and contributes to lowering the blood pressure.

32. Capillary Dynamics

What is the major determinant of blood flow in capillaries?

Blood flow is dependent on the contractile state of the arterioles.

Which processes govern movement of substances across capillaries?

- Diffusion.
- Filtration.
- Pinocytosis.

How is the hydrostatic pressure within the capillary determined?

This depends on arterial pressure, post-capillary venous pressure and the tone of pre- and post-capillary sphincters. Increase in arterial or venous pressure increases hydrostatic pressure. Increase in sphincter tone lowers hydrostatic pressure.

Which is the major force retaining fluid within the capillary?

This is colloid osmotic pressure exerted by the plasma proteins that are retained within the capillary.

How does the interplay between hydrostatic and oncotic pressures determine net fluid movement across the capillary?

This can be represented by Starling's law:

Fluid movement = $k[P_c + \pi_i) - (P_i + \pi_p)]$

where
k = Filtration constant for capillary membrane.
P_c = Capillary hydrostatic pressure.
π_i = Interstitial fluid oncotic pressure.
P_i = Interstitial fluid hydrostatic pressure.
π_p = Plasma protein oncotic pressure.

If the net figure is positive filtration out of the capillary occurs, if negative absorption into the capillary takes place.

33. Valsalva manoeuvre

What is valsalva manoeuvre?

Sustained expiratory effort against a closed glottis, i.e. a sustained increase intrathoracic pressure against a closed or occluded glottis.

Can you give some examples?

- Voluntary increased abdominal pressure against a closed glottis.
- Coughing.
- Mechanically induced by an anaesthetist in a ventilated patient.

What happens to SBP as a result of a voluntarily induced valsalva manoeuvre?

At the initiation of the manoeuvre there is an initial increase, followed by a decease back towards normal. At the end of the manoeuvre there is another transient increase in SBP.

Can you explain these changes?

- Initial rise in SBP: due to compression of the abdominal aorta by voluntary straining.
- Reuction in systolic back towards normal: sustained pressure on the inferior vena cava results in reduced venous return and, due to the Frank–Starling relationship, there is a reduced CO. As blood pressure = cardiac output × total peripheral resistance (BP = CO × TPR) there is a reduction in blood pressure.
- Rise in systolic at the end of the manoeuvre: release of pressure on the inferior vena cava increases venous return and, therefore, for the same reasons outlined above, an increase in CO and SBP.

What happens to the heart rate and systemic vascular resistance during the valsalva manoeuvre?

They both increase steadily.

Can you explain this?

Reduced venous return due to pressure on the inferior vena cava results in a reduced CO (Frank–Starling relationship). This results in a reduction in baroreceptor stimulation and, therefore, an increase in sympathetic outflow to the heart and peripheral vasculature.

34. Control of Respiration

Where are the respiratory centres?
Respiratory centres are located in the pons and the medulla.

What are the main sensors controlling respiration?
The main sensors are the central and peripheral chemoreceptors. Central chemoreceptors are situated on the ventral surface of the medulla and are sensitive to fluctuations in the pH of the cerebrospinal fluid (CSF). Peripheral chemoreceptors are situated in the carotid bodies and aortic arch and are primarily sensitive to fluctuations in PaO_2. There are also mechanical receptors in the lungs and in muscles which help regulate respiration.

How do fluctuations of CSF pH relate to respiration?
Unlike H^+ ions, CO_2 readily crosses the blood–brain barrier. As PCO_2 rises in the periphery it crosses into the CSF and results in an increase in H^+ ion formation, thereby stimulating the central chemoreceptors.

What is the most important determinant of respiratory control?
$PaCO_2$ is the most important factor in controlling respiration. Increases in $PaCO_2$ leads to increases in respiration.

What is the main control of respiration in longstanding lung disease?
In longstanding lung disease, changes in CSF pH compensate for the rise in H^+ and after a prolonged period the central chemoreceptors reset. When this has happened the main drive for respiration is PaO_2 detected by the peripheral chemoreceptors.

35. Lung Volumes and Capacities

What is meant by tidal volume?
The volume of air entering/leaving the lungs during normal inspiration/expiration.

What is meant by forced vital capacity?
The volume of air expelled by maximal expiration following full maximal inspiration.

What is meant by functional residual capacity?
The volume of air left in the lungs following normal tidal expiration.

What is meant by expiratory reserve volume?
The volume of air left in the lungs following maximal expiration.

What is the FEV1/FVC ratio and why is it useful?
It is the ratio of forced expiratory volume in one second over the total forced vital capacity. In a normal subject this ratio is 0.8. It provides a useful way of distinguishing restrictive lung disease (FEV1/FVC > 0.8) from obstructive lung disease (FEV1/FVC < 0.8).

What is the difference between anatomical and physiological dead space?
Anatomical dead space is the portion the tidal volume that remains in the upper part of the respiratory tree that is not involved in gas exchange. Physiological dead space, however, includes all non-exchanging parts of the respiratory tree, i.e. anatomical dead space and alveoli not taking part in gaseous exchange.

36. Pulmonary Dynamics

What do you understand by the terms compliance and hysteresis?
They are both measures of the change in lung volume per unit change in pressure ($\Delta V/\Delta P$) during the breathing cycle. They are, therefore, measures of the degree of elasticity of the lungs. Compliance is measure of lung elasticity as the lung inflates, whereas hysteresis is a measure of lung elasticity as the lung deflates.

Why are the values of compliance and hysteresis different in the same lung?
This is a direct result of the action of surfactant (a detergent-like substance rich in lecithin) which lowers alveolar surface tension and decreases the work of breathing.

What are the implications of this difference when making pressure–volume measurements in the lung?
The volume of the lung at any given pressure will be greater if measured during expiration than if measured during inspiration. This results in the classic pressure–volume loops.

What is meant by the term "work of breathing"?

To expand the lung the inspiratory muscles must overcome the elastic recoil of the lungs and the resistance of the airways to flow.

Is there any way of measuring this work?

Yes, by measuring intrapleural pressure.

37. Pulmonary Gas Exchange and Blood Gas Transport

How is oxygen transported?

Oxygen is carried in two ways:

1. Attached to haemoglobin.
2. As dissolved oxygen in the blood.

What barriers must oxygen traverse to pass from the air in the alveolus to attach to haemoglobin?

- Surfactant.
- Plasmalemma of alveolar epithelium (outer surface of epithelium).
- Cytoplasm of alveolar epithelium.
- Plasmalemma of alveolar epithelium (inner surface of epithelium).
- Basement membrane of epithelium.
- Interstitium.
- Basement membrane of endothelium.
- Plasmalemma of endothelium (outer surface of endothelium).
- Cytoplasm of endothelium.
- Plasmalemma of endothelium (inner surface of endothelium).
- Plasma.
- Plasmalemma of red erythrocyte.
- Cytoplasm of erythrocyte.

What do you understand by impairment of diffusion?

Impaired equilibrium between the alveolar gas and the capillary blood.

What diseases can cause impaired diffusion of oxygen?

Asbestosis, sarcoidosis and interstitial fibrosis.

What shape is the oxygen dissociation curve?

Sigmoidal.

What factors affect the affinity of haemoglobin for oxygen?

H^+, PCO_2, temperature and 2,3-diphosphoglycerate: a rise of any of these factors reduce the affinity of haemoglobin for oxygen and will result in a rightward shift of the oxygen–haemoglobin dissociation curve.

What is the Bohr effect?

As the pH of blood decreases its affinity for oxygen decreases, this is related to deoxygenated haemoglobin having a greater affinity for H^+ than oxyhaemoglobin.

How is carbon dioxide transported in the blood?

It is transported in three ways:

1. Dissolved carbon dioxide.
2. As bicarbonate.
3. Combined with proteins.

Critical Care

AIRWAY ISSUES

BREATHING AND VENTILATION

CIRCULATION AND PERFUSION

HEAD INJURY

SEPSIS

OTHER ISSUES

1. Airway Obstruction

How would you define airway obstruction?

Partial or complete occlusion of the upper or lower respiratory tract, upper airway obstruction being more common than obstruction below the larynx.

In what situations does it occur?

Upper airway obstruction commonly occurs in the unconscious patient who is unable to maintain there airway due to the tongue falling backward. Other causes of upper airway obstruction include: laryngospasm, tumours, soft tissue swellings, oedema, infection (epiglottitis and diphtheria) and foreign objects as well as blood and vomit. In anaesthesia; lower airway obstruction may occur due to pulmonary secretions or mucus plugging, pulmonary oedema, pneumothorax or haemothorax.

What are the clinical features of airway obstruction?

- Hypoventilation.
- Increased work of breathing: accessory muscles of breathing are often employed, tracheal tug may be seen, see-saw paradoxical movement of the abdomen and the chest may also be noticeable.
- Change in noise of breathing: complete obstruction is silent; partial obstruction is noisy (e.g. stridor).
- Tachypnioea.
- Tachycardia.
- Lower respiratory signs will be present if there is lower airway obstruction, but this will depend on the cause of the lower airway obstruction.

How would you clinically assess an airway?

- Look: for accessory muscle movements, see-saw movements of abdomen and chest, foreign bodies in airway; and in late stages central cyanosis.
- Listen: for breath sounds, stridor, grunting and gurgling.
- Feel: for airflow at the nose and mouth; chest movement.

What are the immediate management possibilities?

- Suction/finger sweep: to remove secretions and debris.
- Chin lift or jaw thrust (safest in trauma).
- Airway adjuncts: oro/nasopharyngeal airway.

- Definitive airway: orotracheal intubation, nasotracheal intubation and surgical airway.
- Oxygen therapy.

Are there any contraindications to the airway adjuncts?

- Oropharyngeal airway should not be used in patients with a gag reflex.
- Nasopharyngeal airway should not be used in patients with suspected basal skull fracture.

2. Tracheostomy

What are the indications for tracheostomy?

- A definitive airway is required but orotracheal and nasotracheal intubation is not possible.
- Prolonged intubation is required.

What type of tracheostomy is most commonly performed in the intensive care unit setting?

Percutaneous tracheostomy as this is less traumatic and can be performed with transfer to theatre.

How soon after a tracheostomy should the tube be changed and why?

No sooner than 3 days as it takes this long for a fistula to form so that replacement may be done safely.

How should a tracheostomy be maintained?

The tracheostomy site needs to kept clean to avoid infection. Humidified oxygen should be used and regular tracheal suction will be necessary.

What are the potential complications of a tracheostomy?

- Haemorrhage at the time of insertion.
- Infection.
- Misplacement.
- Blockage.
- Tracheo-oesophageal fistula.

3. Post-operative Hypoxia

Can you describe the respiratory mechanisms that lead to post-operative hypoxia?
- Basal/dependent atelectasis leads to impaired gas exchange.
- Drugs such as opioids suppress ventilatory drive.
- Inadequate pain relief can impair ability to cough leading to retained secretions and respiratory infections.

What are the post-operative strategies used to prevent respiratory complications such as bronchopneumonia?
- Adequate analgesia including epidurals and intercostal blocks.
- Encourage deep breathing and coughing.
- Physiotherapy: chest percussion and postural drainage.
- Early use of antibiotics if there is strong suspicion of infection.

Apart from infection, can you name a few other respiratory causes of post-operative hypoxia?
- Chronic obstructive airways disease.
- Asthma.
- Pleural effusions.
- Pulmonary embolism.
- Pneumothorax.
- Adult respiratory distress syndrome (ARDS).

What investigations would you consider for the hypoxic patient?
- Pulse oximetry.
- Peak-expiratory flow rate (PEFR).
- Arterial blood gases.
- Full blood count.
- Chest radiograph.
- Electrocardiography.
- Sputum microscopy and culture.

What methods are available to provide oxygen for the hypoxic patient?
- Oxygen by face mask or nasal prongs.
- Continuous positive airway pressure.
- Non-invasive positive pressure ventilation (NIPPV).
- Intubation and ventilation.

4. Respiratory Failure and Blood-Gas Analysis

Can you list some causes of respiratory failure where the $PaCO_2$ is raised?

- Depression of respiratory centre: sedatives, trauma and raised intracranial pressure.
- Chest wall problem: flail chest and kyphoscoliosis.
- Neuromuscular disease: Guillain–Barré and poliomyelitis.
- Severe obstructive airways disease.

Can you do the same for instances where $PaCO_2$ is reduced or normal?

- Collapse/consolidation (e.g. pneumonia).
- Pulmonary contusion.
- Asthma.
- Cardiac disease (e.g. left ventricular failure).
- Pulmonary embolism.

What are the signs of impending respiratory arrest?

- Respiratory rate >30.
- Tachycardia >120.
- Hypotension.
- Sympathetic activation: sweaty, clammy and agitated.
- Fall in PaO_2.
- Rapid desaturation when oxygen withdrawn.

The following arterial blood gas results were obtained from a young man with an isolated chest injury following a road traffic accident. Can you comment?

- PH: 7.24.
- PaO_2: 8 kPa.
- $PaCO_2$: 9 kPa.
- Bicarbonate: 29 mmol/l.

There is an acidosis and the raised $PaCO_2$ suggests that this is respiratory in origin. The low PaO_2 with a raised $PaCO_2$ could be explained by hypoventilation secondary to a large flail chest injury.

What is the definition of base excess obtained from blood-gas analysis?

This is the amount of acid (mmol) required to restore 1 l of blood to normal pH at 37°C and PCO_2 of 5.3 kPa. Normal range is −2 to +2 mmol/l.

5. Artificial Ventilation

Can you name some indications for mechanical ventilation?

- Correction of hypoxia/hypercapnia in respiratory failure.
- Protect the airway in the "drowsy" patient (Glasgow coma scale, GCS <8).
- Allow effective suctioning of respiratory secretions.
- To improve oxygen delivery to tissues.

What is non-invasive ventilation?

This does not require intubation but employs a face mask to provide ventilatory assistance with breathing (spontaneous pressure support) or to deliver timed breaths (pressure controlled ventilation). A valve employed for the exhalation cycle reduces rebreathing. This method of ventilation is useful for conditions such as chronic obstructive airways disease.

What are the principles of methods of assisted ventilation such as synchronised intermittent mandatory ventilation (SIMV)?

These methods allow spontaneous respiratory effort by the patient to contribute to the ventilatory process. A predetermined tidal volume and frequency of breathing is set on the machine. If there is no respiratory effort from the patient then the machine delivers a breath of the preset parameters. However, if the patient attempts to breath alone the number of machine delivered breaths is reduced, allowing the patient to "fill in the gaps".

How is the patient weaned from artificial ventilation?

Gradual and progressive reduction of support can be initiated using SIMV as outlined above. Alternatively, the patient may be disconnected from the ventilator for increasing periods of time to allow spontaneous respiration. The capability to cough effectively is essential before extubation.

Can you name some complications of artificial ventilation?

- Related to the airway: trauma from endotracheal tube or tracheostomy, misplaced endotracheal tube and hypotension during intubation.
- Ventilator-induced lung injury (e.g. pnuemothorax).
- Ventilator-associated pneumonia.

- Hyotension secondary to positive intrathoracic pressure reducing venous return to heart.
- Inadvertent disconnection from the ventilator.

6. Adult Respiratory Distress Syndrome

What are the criteria for diagnosis of ARDS?
- Bilateral pulmonary infiltrates on chest X-ray.
- PaO_2/FiO_2 ratio <200.
- Pulmonary artery wedge pressure <18 mmHg.

What are the causes of ARDS?
Systemic
- Sepsis.
- Trauma.
- Burns.
- Massive blood transfusion.
- Post-cardiac arrest.
- Pancreatitis.
- Anaphylactic shock.

Pulmonary
- Lung infections.
- Pulmonary trauma.
- Smoke inhalation.
- Near drowning.
- Aspiration.

What is the pathophysiology of ARDS?
The localised or systemic insult results in release of interleukins (e.g. IL-1, 6, and 8) and tumour necrosis factor α (TNFα). These mediators cause white cell activation, adhesion and migration from peri-alveolar capillaries into alveoli. In addition, endothelial and alveolar cell damage results in increased permeability, pulmonary oedema and alveolar collapse.

What are the aims of mechanical ventilation for ARDS?
- Prevent alveolar collapse and recruit collapsed alveoli by using high positive end-expiratory pressures.
- Use low tidal volumes and low peak inspiratory pressures to reduce lung damage that may be caused by ventilation.

What is the mortality from ARDS?

This depends on underlying cause, age of patient. When the under-lying cause is trauma mortality is typically 30–40%. When ARDS is secondary to sepsis mortality is around 60%. However, the highest mortality for ARDS is when it occurs secondary to aspiration pneu-monia when the mortality is 90%.

Breathing and Ventilation

CIRCULATION AND PERFUSION

7. Heart Failure

What are the symptoms and signs of heart failure?
Symptoms
- Shortness of breath at rest or on minimal exertion.
- Orthopnoea.
- Paroxysmal nocturnal dyspnoea.

Signs
- Third heart sound.
- Raised Jugular venous pressure (JVP).
- Peripheral oedema.
- Displaced apex beat.
- Basal crepitations.
- Pulsus alternans.

What can be done pre-operatively to assess fitness for surgery in someone with heart failure ?
History and physical examination are always the first part of the assessment. An electrocardiography (ECG) and chest X-ray are easily arranged first-line investigations. Echocardiography is extremely useful as a left ventricular ejection fraction of <35% is associated with high risk of peri-operative myocardial infarction (MI). Liaison with a cardiologist may be necessary.

What cardiovascular effects can general anaesthetics have?
- Changes in the arterial and central venous pressure (CVP).
- Reduce systemic vascular resistance (SVR).
- Reduce myocardial contractility (and hence reduce stroke volume).
- Increase myocardial irritability.

Note: Fentanyl causes less cardiac depression than many other general anaesthetic agents but it still has an effect on venodilatation which reduces preload and hence cardiac output (CO). Patients with congestive heart failure are very sensitive to this effect.

What other anaesthetic options are there for patients with congestive heart failure?
Epidural and spinal anaesthesia can be used. However, both these methods still cause venodilatation by blocking sympathetic outflow,

decreasing preload and therefore reducing CO. It is possible to increase preload by administering fluids pre-operatively but this increases the post-operative risk of heart failure. Recent studies comparing general and regional anaesthesia found that there may be no difference in cardiac complications or mortality.

How would you classify the risks for surgical procedures with respect to the likelihood of cardiac complications?

- High risk (>5% risk of peri-operative death or MI): aortic surgery; peripheral vascular surgery; or prolonged procedures of the abdomen, head or thorax.
- Intermediate risk (1–5% risk of peri-operative mortality or MI): orthopaedic or urological surgery.
- Low risk (<1% risk of peri-operative mortality or MI): endoscopy and cataract surgery.

8. Cardiac Arrest

What types of cardiac arrest do you know?

Cardiac arrests are classified into: ventricular fibrillation (VF) arrests, pulseless electrical activity (PEA) arrests and asystolic arrests.

What interventions have been found to improve survival in cardiac arrest?

Early defibrillation: the probability of successful defibrillation decreases by approximately 5% every minute from the onset of the arrest.

Basic life support: respiratory support and cardiac massage delay the onset of asystole in a VF or PEA arrest.

Does this mean all other components of the cardiac arrest algorithm are worthless?

No, it is just difficult to design studies to examine the effects of any single interventions in cardiac arrest patients.

What drugs do you know that are used in a cardiac arrest situation?

- Adrenaline.
- Atropine.
- Lignocaine.
- Calcium chloride.
- Sodium bicarbonate.

How should these drugs be administered ideally in a cardiac arrest situation?

Ideally, these drugs should be administered by a central vein. However, peripheral canulae are most commonly used and some drugs (adrenaline and atropine) can be given endotracheally if no intravenous (i.v.) access is available.

What is the effect of adrenaline in cardiac arrest?

It helps maintain coronary and cerebral perfusion through its α constrictor effects.

9. Principles of Cardiovascular Monitoring

What non-invasive means of cardiovascular monitoring do you know?

The lead II ECG shows heart rate and rhythm. The pulse oximeter monitors arterial blood oxygen saturation and heart rate. Blood pressure can be measured using an automated sphygmomanometer.

What are the pitfalls of using a pulse oximeter?

A pulse oximeter does not measure the ability to blow off carbon dioxide. So a patient may have inadequate alveolar ventilation, despite SaO_2 of 100%. Pulse oximetry does not warn against reductions in tissue oxygen delivery, caused by anaemia or poor CO. Pulse oximetry is indeed inaccurate when tissue perfusion is poor, because of vasoconstriction. Saturations <70% are calculated, not measured, and may be erroneous.

What invasive means of cardiovascular monitoring do you know?

An arterial line can be used to directly measure blood pressure. Catheters may be used to measure either CVP or pulmonary artery wedge pressure (PAWP). A transoesophageal Doppler probe can estimate CO.

What are the problems and complications of arterial pressure monitoring?

- Over- and under-dampening which may be due to a clot, air bubbles or a very compliant diaphragm and tube.
- Incorrect zeroing: the transducer must be placed at the level of the right atrium.
- Haematoma and distal ischaemia.
- Arterial thrombus.

- Inadvertent drug injection.
- Disconnection and haemorrhage.
- Infection.

What are the complications of central venous access?
- Arterial puncture and trauma.
- Pneumothorax.
- Haemothorax.
- Air embolism.
- Haematoma.
- Catheter embolism.
- Dysrhythmias.
- Cardiac perforation and tamponade.
- Damage to surrounding structures (e.g. thoracic duct, trachea and thyroid).
- Infection (local, bacteraemia and endocarditis).

10. Swan–Ganz Catheters

What do you use a Swan–Ganz catheter for?
A Swan–Ganz catheter measures pressures in the pulmonary artery and, indirectly, left heart filling pressure. Blood can be aspirated from its ports to measure saturations in the right atrium and right ventricle. It can also be used to measure CO and estimate SVR.

What are the indications for inserting a Swan–Ganz catheter?
- Measurement of PAWP to assess fluid status and optimise CO: oliguria, hypotension, right ventricular infarction, shock, adult respiratory distress syndrome (ARDS) to differentiate between cardiac and non-cardiac pulmonary oedema.
- Measurement of CO and SVR to guide inotropic therapy in shock.
- Measurement of right heart blood SaO_2 to diagnose of left to right shunts.

How do you place a Swan–Ganz catheter?
The inflated balloon on the catheter's tip lets it float in the lumen. As the Swan–Ganz catheter is advanced through the right heart, the pressure tracings from its tip identify where it is (right atrium, right ventricle and pulmonary artery). Advancing the catheter further causes it to "wedge" in the pulmonary artery. The balloon should always be deflated between PAWP measurements. The tracing during the insertion of a Swan–Ganz catheter is shown in Figure 7.

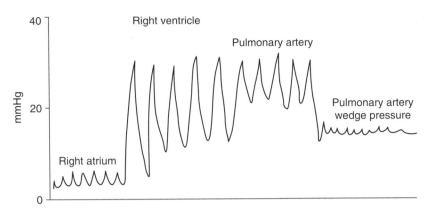

Figure 7 Tracing during insertion of a Swan–Ganz catheter.

What are the complications of inserting a Swan–Ganz catheter?
- Complications of central venous cannulation (as outlined above).
- Dysrhythmias.
- Heart block.
- Valvular damage.
- Perforation.
- Knotting.
- Thrombosis.
- Pulmonary infarction.
- Arterial laceration.

How do you measure CO using a Swan–Ganz catheter?
CO can be measured using thermodilution. A known volume of cold saline (between 4°C and room temperature) is injected into the right atrium via proximal port of the catheter. A thermistor at the tip of the catheter measures the resulting drop in the temperature of the blood. A plot of temperature change against time gives a curve from which of CO can be calculated from the area under the curve.

Why is the clinical use of Swan–Ganz catheters controversial?
The controversy of the use of Swan–Ganz catheters arose because studies in the mid-1990s found that patients who received a Swan–Ganz catheter had a higher mortality than patients who did not receive a Swan–Ganz catheter. However, it was argued that patients who received Swan–Ganz catheters were, by definition, sicker than those for who they are not indicated, therefore patients receiving Swan–Ganz catheters were more likely to have a greater mortality. Further studies, including meta-analyses of randomised

controlled trials on Swan–Ganz-guided strategies found a modest risk reduction in mortality: the risk reduction appeared greatest in surgical patients. There are still no consensus guidelines for clinical practice.

11. Shock

What do you understand by the term "shock"?
Shock is inadequate tissue oxygenation because of a failure of the circulatory system.

What different types of shock do you know of?
The failure of the circulatory system may be due to pump failure (cardiogenic shock), hypovolaemia (hypovolaemic shock) or excessive peripheral vasodilatation.

Can you give some example causes of each type of shock?
Cardiogenic shock
- MI/ischaemia.
- Dysrhythmias.
- Pulmonary embolism.
- Cardiac tamponade.
- Tension pneumothorax.

Hypovolaemic shock
- Haemorrhage.
- Gastro-intestinal fluid loss.
- Burns.
- Third-space sequestration.

Vasodilatation
- Sepsis.
- Drugs and poisons.
- Anaphylaxis.
- Spinal cord injury/anaesthesia.

How do you assess volume status in a patient with suspected shock?
Examine the patient for signs of hypovolaemia or fluid overload: pulse and blood pressure (especially postural drop), JVP, basal crackles (interstitial compartment), peripheral perfusion (e.g. capillary refill) and oedema (interstitial compartment). The charts should be checked for serial weights and fluid balance (input/output). Additional tools

include chest X-rays (signs of pulmonary oedema or cardiomegaly), a CVP line (used dynamically) and a Swan–Ganz catheter.

How can a Swan–Ganz catheter help in the diagnosis of shock?

The calculation of PAWP, CO and SVR is used to diagnose shock. A high PAWP, low CO and high SVR is consistent with cardiogenic shock. A low PAWP, high CO and low SVR is characteristic of septic shock. However, these are not absolute. For example in profound sepsis, myocardial depression also occurs due to circulating cytokines such as tumour necrosis factor (TNF).

12. Inotropes

How do you assess the need for inotropes?

If there is hypotension in the face of a high PAWP, which implies fluid overload or cardiogenic shock, or if hypotension persists despite correcting hypovolaemia, then inotropes are indicated.

What are the pharmacological mechanisms of action of inotropes work?

Inotropes increase myocardial contractility in a variety of ways. For example, digoxin increases intracellular calcium stores in the myocardium. Catecholamines stimulate the myocardium through their action on β_1 receptors on the surface of myocardial cells. Others may act indirectly, e.g. dopexamine increases the level of endogenous noradrenaline by inhibiting its neuronal re-uptake.

Apart from their effect on myocardial contractility, is there any other effect of inotropes that is important to know about when selecting the appropriate one to use?

Yes, inotropes also affect the peripheral vasculature in different ways, e.g. adrenaline and noradrenaline both have β_1 inotropic effects but adrenaline has β_2 vasoldilatory and α_1 vasoconstrictor effects in the periphery, whereas noradrenaline only has α_1 constrictor effects in the periphery. Similarly, dobutamine is a β_2 vasodilator, whereas dopamine is an α_1 vasoconstrictor. However, it is important to realise that these receptor profiles are dose dependent. Adrenaline has exhibits β_2 vasodilatory effects at a lower dose than it has α_1 vasoconstrictor effects, and dopamine exhibits α_1 vasoconstrictor effects at much higher dose than its β_1 intotropic effects.

What inotrope would you use in cardiogenic shock due to left ventricular failure?

Dopamine.

What inotrope would you use in cardiogenic shock due to pulmonary embolism?

Noradrenaline.

What inotrope would you use in septic shock?

Noradrenaline.

What inotrope would you use in anaphylactic shock?

Adrenaline.

13. Management of Head Injury

What are the immediate priorities in managing a patient who is comatose due to a head injury?

The priorities are those outlined in the advanced trauma life support (ATLS) guidelines. Attention should be given to support of airway (and cervical spine protection), breathing and circulation.

Consider a patient who is comatose after head injury. After adequate resuscitation a computed tomography head scan is performed and the patient is found to have not to have any intracranial haematomas or focal contusions. What is the likely reason for the coma?

It is likely that the patient has suffered a diffuse axonal injury. However, it is important to investigate and treat other possible causes for the coma, e.g. fits or electrolyte abnormalities.

Consider a 22-year old male who has suffered a head injury but is fully conscious after a brief period of coma (minutes). A computed tomography head scan reveals the presence of small bilateral frontal contusions. The patient lives at home with his family who say they are able to look after him. Should this patient be admitted to hospital?

Yes. The contusions may blossom over the next 72 hours resulting in deterioration in the patient's condition. Supportive care and/or an operation may then be required.

What are the aims of management of the head-injured patient?

The first aim is to protect the brain from further damage as secondary brain damage may result from ischaemia due to fluctuation is blood pressure or due to further development of the primary lesion, e.g. further swelling around areas of contusion. In addition, head-injured patients often have associated injuries, e.g. cervical spine and limb injuries which need to be investigated and treated.

What metabolic abnormality common in head injuries is associated with a poor prognosis?

Diabetes insipidus.

Should steroids be used routinely in the management of head-injured patients?

No. There is no evidence that outcome from head injury is improved by the use of high dose steroids. However, this situation may change depending on the results of on-going trials.

14. Control of Intracranial Pressure

What is the Munro–Kelly hypothesis?

The Munro–Kelly hypothesis (1852) postulated that the intracranial contents (blood, cerebrospinal fluid (CSF) and brain tissue) are not compressible and thus an increase in volume of any part causes a rapid increase in pressure.

Can you give the normal range of intracranial pressure (ICP) values for a healthy individual?

The range is 0–10 mmHg.

Why should we be concerned about an elevated ICP?

Raised ICP will reduce cerebral perfusion with a resulting risk of ischaemic damage to brain cells.

What values of ICP should we be concerned about?

An ICP of >15 mmHg over a sustained period is termed "intracranial hypertension" although cerebral ishcaemia is unlikely to occur in this range. An ICP of >20 mmHg is associated with areas of focal ischaemia and ICPs >50 mmHg will result in global ischaemia.

What is the relation between cerebral perfusion pressure (CPP) and ICP and what are the implications of this relationship for the management of ICP?

CPP is the difference between the mean arterial pressure (MAP) and ICP, i.e. CPP = MAP − ICP. In practice a CPP of 70 mmHg is aimed for so that if there is a raised ICP the MAP can be increased accordingly, e.g. with inotropes. However, if there is impairment of the normal autoregulatory mechanisms, maintaining an adequate CPP will not necessarily prevent focal or global ischaemia.

In an unconscious patient, how is ICP measured?

ICP is usually measured through an extracranial transducer connected to a ventricular catheter or subdural bolt.

If the ICP was not being measured, what features would point towards a raised ICP in an unconscious patient?

The presence of the Cushing reflex (rising blood pressure with associated bradycardia), or evidence of coning (dilated pupil or pupils and/or posturing).

What factors may contribute to a raised ICP?

- Intracranial lesions, e.g. tumour and blood clot (traumatic or spontaneous bleed from an aneurysm).
- Brain swelling secondary to primary lesion (this may be delayed, e.g. blossoming of a traumatic contusion or oedema around a tumour).
- Hyperthermia.
- Hyperglycaemia.
- Hypercarbia.
- Raised venous pressure.
- Hypermetabolism.

Can you briefly describe ways in which an ICP of >40 mmHg might be treated in a patient with a diffuse head injury with no intracranial blood clots?

1. Diuresis with mannitol.
2. Maintain PCO_2 in the 4.5–5 kPa range: an overly raised PCO_2 produces vasodilation and increases ICP and reduced PCO_2 reduces ICP by producing vasoconstriction (this is the Munro–Kelly hypothesis). However, too low a PCO_2 may produce ischaemia due to too much vasoconstriction.
3. Control any seizures to help reduce metabolic rate (may need to paralyse patient pharmacologically).
4. Reduce the temperature of patient to normothermic or slightly hypothermic.
5. Thiopentone can be considered but is controversial.
6. Consider decompressive craniectomy.

What types of coning do you know about?

There are essentially two types of coning: transtentorial and central.

- Transtentorial coning can be in a downward direction due the temporal lobe uncus pressing on the brainstem resulting ipsilteral third nerve palsy, Cushing reflex and decerebrate drigidity. It can also occur in an upward direction is there is a posterior fossa mass or bleed pushing cerebellar tissue up through the tentorial incisura.
- Central coning occurs when there is herniation of the cerebellum and medulla down through the foramen magnum resulting in Cheyne–Stokes breathing, sudden apnoea and neck stiffness.

15. Brainstem Death

Who should undertake brainstem function testing?
Two doctors who have been qualified for at least 5 years.

What are the criteria for brainstem death?
1. Absence of anaesthesia (sedatives or parlaysing agents).
2. Normothermia.
3. Normal blood biochemistry.
4. No motor response to painful stimuli.
5. No pupillary light reflex.
6. No corneal reflex.
7. Absent Doll's eye reflex.
8. Negative caloric testing.
9. No gag reflex.
10. Absence of respiratory effort.

Are there any conditions that must be satisfied before brainstem testing can be undertaken?
Yes, the patient must have a diagnosis compatible with brainstem death and have been in a coma for at least 6 hours.

Are there any investigations that might be used to help confirm brainstem death?
Electroencephalogram (EEG) testing may be used.

SEPSIS

16. Terminology

What is an infection?
The invasion of a host by micro-organisms resulting in an inflammatory response.

What is the difference between bacteraemia and septicaemia?
Both bacteraemia and septicaemia are characterised by the presence of viable bacteria in the blood. However, septicaemia is associated with a systemic response.

What are the criteria which define sepsis?
Sepsis is a systemic response to infection characterised by at least two of the following criteria: temperature >38°C or <36°C, heart rate >90/minute, respiratory rate >20 breaths/minute (or $PaCO_2$ < 32 mmHg), white cell count >12,000 cells/mm^3 (or <4000 cells/mm^3, or >10% immature forms).

What is the difference between sepsis and septic shock?
Septic shock is the state sepsis but with associated hypotension despite adequate fluid resuscitation.

17. Consequences of Sepsis

Gram-negative septicaemia can have life-threatening consequences. How do these organisms cause such severe pathology?
Gram-negative rods have a lipopolysaccharide (LPS) in their cell wall, which is a powerful endotoxin. LPS activates a wide range of inflammatory cascades.

Name some of the inflammatory mediators involved.
- Tumour necrosis factor (TNF).
- Interleukins.
- Prostaglandins leucotriens.
- Nitric oxide.
- Bradykinin.
- Complement.

How do these mediators lead to septic shock?

The effect of these inflammatory cascades is to increase the body's metabolic needs and cause massive vasodilatation. The systemic vascular resistance (SVR) falls precipitously and hypotension results despite increased cardiac output. This results in the classic appearance of septic shock of an unwell, hypotensive patient with flushed cheeks, warm peripheries and bounding pulses.

What other organ systems are affected by these inflammatory cascades?

- Haematological: clotting cascade activated, micro clots and bleeding as factors consumed. This is disseminated intravascular coagulopathy (DIC).
- Respiratory: inflammatory mediators lead to leaky capillaries and adult respiratory distress syndrome (ARDS).
- Neurological: poor perfusion leads to confusion, drowsiness and coma.
- Cardiac: increased work can result in ischaemia and failure in end stage shock.
- Renal: mediators and poor perfusion lead to acute tubular necrosis (ATN).
- Hepatic: liver failure can result from hypotension.
- Intestinal: ischaemic bowel becomes permeable to bacteria leading to translocation and further septic insult.

How is this clinical picture labelled?

This is labelled as multi-organ dysfunction syndrome (MODS).

What is the prognosis?

Prognosis is poor, mortality approaches 95% with established three-organ failure.

18. Principles of Sepsis Management

What are the principles of treating sepsis?

- Resuscitate/supportive therapy with appropriate monitoring.
- Remove source of sepsis/drain pus.
- Appropriate antibiotics, as narrow spectrum as is safe.

What needs to be considered before starting antibiotics?

- Have appropriate cultures been sent?
- Will the antibiotic cover the most likely organisms (local policy useful)? Broad-spectrum antibiotics can be used if there is no time to wait for cultures.

What is the mainstay of supportive therapy in sepsis?

- Fluid resuscitation.
- Vasopressors.
- Organ support as required.
- Monitoring.

By what means can the source of sepsis be removed/drained?

- Incise and drain abscess.
- Debride infected tissue (trauma/necrotising fascitis).
- Amputation (gangrenous limb).
- Percutaneous/open drainage of collection.

Do you know of any specific treatment that is acquiring an evidence base?

Anti-protein C, an exciting development as previous immune modulators have failed in trials.

19. Sources of Sepsis

List some categories of infection in a surgical patient?

- Wound infection.
- Pneumonia.
- Urinary tract infection (UTI).
- Bacteraemia from intravascular devices.

What are the broad sources of bacterial infection? Where can it arise?

Endogenous and exogenous organisms.

Can you explain these terms?

- Endogenous infections arise form the patient's own flora.
- Exogenous micro-organisms come from elsewhere: the air, medical equipment, the surgeon or other health care workers.

In broad terms, what factors predispose to an endogenous wound infection?

These can be summarised by remembering that:

$$\text{Risk of infection} = \frac{\text{Dose of bacteria} \times \text{Virulence}}{\text{Patient resistance}}$$

What effects patient resistance?

- Age.
- Nutrition.
- Obesity.
- Diabetes.
- Smoking.
- Immunosuppression.
- Malignancy.
- Renal failure.
- Anaemia.
- Jaundice.

What factors during the operation increase the risk of surgical site infection?

- Inadequate skin preparation.
- Pre-operative shaving.
- Long procedure.
- Foreign material.
- Drains.
- Poor haemostasis.
- Tissue trauma.
- Poor sterile technique.

20. Multi-organ dysfunction syndrome

What is multiple organ dysfunction syndrome?

This refers to altered organ function in an acutely ill patient such that homoeostasis cannot be maintained without intervention.

It usually follows a predictable course starting with the lungs progressing to heart, liver, gastro-intestinal tract and kidneys.

What is the mechanism leading to multi-organ dysfunction syndrome (MODS)?

The main causes of MODS are:

- Infection.
- Inflammation, e.g. acute pancreatitis.
- Injury, e.g. trauma and burns.
- Ischaemia.
- Immune.
- Idiopathic.

These triggers initiate an inflammatory response which progresses to multiple organ dysfunction and can lead to death.

Do you know the difference between primary and secondary MODS?

- In primary MODS, a well-defined insult leads directly to organ dysfunction. This injury is severe enough to provoke the systemic inflammatory response syndrome which leads to MODS.
- Secondary MODS develops as a consequence of the host response to the inflammatory response syndrome. "Two hits" are required. The first insult primes the host. The second insult brings about a greatly amplified systemic inflammatory response.

How would you manage a surgical patient at risk of developing MODS?

It is important prior to surgery to predict and anticipate complications to try and prevent a patient going into multi-organ failure.

The aims of treatment are to restore and maintain optimal oxygenation and tissue perfusion. The patient should be treated with high flow oxygen and fluids (colloid or crystalloid).

A careful history and examination is required with review of the patient's medical notes. Appropriate investigations to identify the cause should be carried out. This would include a full blood count and clotting, renal and liver function tests, septic screen, chest X-ray and electrocardiography (ECG). Other modalities of imaging may also be required. Empirical broad-spectrum antibiotics may be started. Operative intervention may be carried out if appropriate.

How would you proceed if the patient develops MODS?

This patient would require management in an intensive care unit (ICU). He may develop adult respiratory distress syndrome and may require ventilatory support. Adequate renal support and antibiotics should be given. It is also important to maintain adequate nutritional support.

Why is it preferable to have enteral feeding in these patients?

Enteral feeding helps to prevent colonisation by pathogenic flora and maintain a mechanical gastro-intestinal mucosal barrier. In addition, enteral feeding maintains gut-associated immunity and blunts the catabolic stress response.

Do you know of any experimental therapies that have been tried to improve outcome in MODS?

Antibodies to tumour necrosis factor α (TNFα), interleukin-8 (IL-8) and endotoxins have been tried with little success.

21. Diabetic Ketoacidosis

What is diabetic ketoacidosis?

Diabetic ketoacidosis is defined as a metabolic acidosis (arterial pH <7.3) associated with ketonaemia and a blood glucose >11 mmol/l.

What are the predisposing factors to diabetic ketoacidosis?

- Surgery.
- Infection.
- Inappropriate reduction of insulin.
- Myocardial infarction.
- Stress.

Can you explain why blood sugar rises in response to surgery?

This occurs as part of the metabolic response to injury. A rise in growth hormone levels decreases glucose uptake in tissues. Increased cortisol levels stimulate gluconeogenesis. Increased levels of cate-cholamines stimulate gluconeogenesis and increased glucagons levels stimulate gluconeogenesis and glycogenolysis. Insulin levels do increase, but this is countered by a degree of insulin resistance, helping maintain a hyperglycaemic state.

What are the clinical features of diabetic ketoacidosis?
- Polyuria.
- Thirst.
- Abdominal pain.
- Vomiting.
- Hyperventilation.
- Hypotension and tachycardia.
- Drowsiness and coma.
- Sweet-smelling ketotic breath.

What are the principles of management?
Diabetic ketoacidosis is a medical emergency. The main principles of management are to replace lost fluid and minerals and administer insulin to counteract the metabolic disturbance. Fluids in the form of normal saline should be given rapidly to try to overcome the fluid deficit. Over the first few hours of treatment, this can then be adjusted according to the patient's clinical condition. Insulin is given as a con-tinuous sliding scale infusion depending on the blood glucose of the patient. Potassium supplements need to be administered as insulin leads to potassium uptake by cells. Further supportive measures such as nasogastric drainage and bladder catheterisation may be required. It may be necessary to transfer the patient to a high-dependency unit (HDU).

22. Burns

How can burns be classified?
They can be classified in terms of the depth of burn into: superficial, partial thickness, (mid-dermal), partial thickness (deep dermal) and full thickness.

What are the pathophysiological features of a burn?
- Increased capillary permeability: this leads to fluid loss, which is proportional to the size and depth of the burn (with large burns, increased plasma loss can lead to hypovolaemic shock).
- Heat loss: loss of normal skin leads to increased evaporation.
- Altered cell metabolism.

What metabolic changes occur with burns?

- Increased metabolic rate.
- Increase in anaerobic metabolism.
- Increased catabolism of proteins.
- Lipolysis.
- Gluconeogenesis: increases in plasma cortisol and catecholamines.
- Impaired insulin release.

Do you know any ways of estimating the area of a burn?

Wallace's rule of nines can be used: head and neck 9%, each arm 9%, anterior trunk 18%, posterior trunk 18%, each leg 18% and perineum 1%.

A more accurate measure can be obtained using Lund and Browder charts which give more accurate proportions for both adults and children.

What would be your immediate management of a burns patient?

The principles of advanced trauma life support (ATLS) must be followed. It is important to know from the history, the time of injury and the cause of the burn with relevant past medical history. It is important to look for evidence of inhalational damage: mucosal redness, soot in upper airway, singed nasal hairs, hoarseness, stridor and difficulty swallowing. An early anaesthetic opinion should be obtained regarding early intubation. An escharotomy may be required if there is a risk to breathing or to the distal circulation of a limb due to constriction of an area of a full thickness burn.

How would you calculate how much fluid needs to be given?

Several formulae are available. A commonly used formula is the Muir and Barclay formula. This calculates the amount of fluid to be given over the first 36 hours.

$$V = \frac{\text{Body weight (kg)} \times \text{Body surface area (\%)}}{2}$$

V is the amount to be given 4 hourly for the first 12 hours, 6 hourly for the next 12 hours and then 12 hourly. This is in addition to the patient's normal fluid requirements.

What are the complications of burns?

Local
- Infection.
- Inhalational injury.
- Ischaemia.
- Scarring and contractures.

Systemic
- Hypovolaemic shock.
- Septicaemia.
- Respiratory insufficiency.
- Renal failure.
- Ileus.
- Haemoglobinuria.
- Curling's ulcer.
- Disseminated intravascular coagulation (DIC).

23. Nutrition

How would you assess the nutritional status of a patient?
- Clinical inspection: appearance through the loss of fat and muscle, and respiratory muscle function.
- Dynamometric: hand grip strength.
- Anthropometric: triceps skinfold thickness, mid-arm muscle circumference and lean body mass.
- Biochemical/haematological: serum proteins (e.g. albumin).

How may nutritional support be delivered?
Enterally or parenterally. Enteral feeding involves introducing feed into the stomach or small bowel. In the stomach, this may be with oral supplements, a nasogastric feeding tube or a gastrostomy tube. In the small bowel, a nasojejunal tube or feeding jejunostomy may be required. Parenteral feeding can be either peripheral, through a long line, or central through a jugular or subclavian line.

Which type of feeding is preferable?
Enteral feeding is preferable to parenteral for a number of reasons because it is more physiological and it helps prevent translocation of gut flora into the blood. In addition, enteral feeding avoids the complications of central line insertion.

What are the indications for enteral feeding?
- Moderate to severe malnutrition with inadequate oral intake.
- Dysphagia.
- Post-head injury.
- Massive enterectomy.
- Distal enterocutaneous fistula.
- Sepsis.

Are there any contraindications to enteral feeding?
- Complete small bowel obstruction.
- Paralytic ileus.
- Proximal small intestinal fistula.
- Severe pancreatitis.

What are the constituents of a parenteral nutrition diet?
- Macronutrients: consisting mainly of energy sources. Many regimens have a combination of 50% carbohydrate and 50% lipid. Nitrogen sources are present as amino acids.
- Micronutrients: vitamins, electrolytes and trace elements.

What are the complications of enteral feeding?
- Fistulae.
- Peritonitis.
- Catheter migration or malposition.
- Tube blockage.
- Aspiration of feed.
- Diarrhoea, nausea, cramps and abdominal bloating.
- Metabolic: electrolyte disturbances and electrolyte abnormalities.

24. Intensive Care Unit Admissions

What parameters would you measure in a seriously ill patient that may help in determining the requirement for ICU?
Many centres have developed an early warning scoring system that measure physiological parameters. These scoring systems help alert junior staff as to whether a patient may require admission to an ICU. Parameters that are particularly useful include: heart rate, blood pressure, respiratory rate, temperature, conscious level, oxygen saturations, urine output and blood pH.

What other factors need to be taken into account in assessing suitability for admission?
The diagnosis and severity of illness need to be taken into account so that maximal benefit can be provided for the right patient. It is important to differentiate between the sick patient for who may have a good prognosis from the moribund patients with a terminal diagnosis. The wishes of the patient and their future quality of life should also be taken into account.

How would you decide if a patient should be admitted to ICU or HDU?

HDU is suitable for patients with impairment of a single organ system who require detailed monitoring but not mechanical ventilatory support. ICU should be reserved for patients who require, or have a high probability of requiring, mechanical ventiltatory support, require detailed and/or invasive monitoring, and have impending multiple organ system failure.

What are the problems in admitting emergency patients to ICU?

These patients are usually older, with often an incomplete knowledge of their past medical history. They are less well optimised for surgery. They may be multiple trauma patients.

25. Scoring Systems in Intensive Care Unit

Why do we have scoring systems in ICU?

Scoring systems provide a means whereby parameters can be measured repeatedly in a relatively easy manner that can be reproduced reliably by different individuals on different occasions. This helps to reduce interobserver variability and allows for more accurate assessments of prognosis and severity of illness. Scoring systems also allow for comparison between units, thereby facilitating audit and research.

What is the most commonly used disease severity scoring system in the UK?

The acute physiology and chronic health evaluation II system (APACHE II).

How is this system used?

It combines 12 physiological parameters with age and chronic health score. Physiological parameters included are: temperature, blood pressure, heart rate, respiratory rate, oxygen therapy required, arterial pH, serum sodium, serum potassium, creatinine, packed cell volume, white blood cell count and neurological score. Data are entered on admission to the ICU and then after 24 hours. The resulting score provides an index of disease severity and a percentage risk of death.

What is the predicted risk of death with an APACHE score of >40?

The risk is 100%.

What other types of scoring system are commonly used in the ICU?

- The Glasgow coma scale (GCS): to score measure conscious level.
- Sedation scores: to help titrate sedation in mechanically ventilated patients.
- Therapeutic intervention scores.
- Injury severity scores.

GROWTH AND DIFFERENTIATION

DEATH, DAMAGE AND DEGENERATION

REGENERATION AND REPAIR

INFLAMMATION AND IMMUNOLOGY

PRINCIPLES OF ONCOLOGY

HAEMATOLOGY

MICROBIOLOGY

1. Hyperplasia and Hypertrophy

Define hypertrophy.
The growth of a tissue or organ because cells increase in size without cell replication.

Define hyperplasia.
The growth of a tissue or organ because there is an increase in the number of cells due to cell division.

Give a physiological and pathological cause of hypertrophy.
Muscles undergo hypertrophy with exercise while cardiomyopathies involve heart muscle hypertrophy.

Give a physiological and pathological cause of hyperplasia.
Hyperplasia takes place in the breast during puberty and pregnancy while adrenal hyperplasia characterises Cushing's disease.

Can you name any conditions in which hypertrophy and hyperplasia occur in the same organ?
- Benign prostatic enlargement.
- Grave's disease of the thyroid.

What is autonomous hyperplasia?
Proliferation in the absence of a demonstrable stimulus as in psoriasis and Paget's disease of bone. This falls very close to the definition of neoplasia.

2. Metaplasia

Define metaplasia.
The reversible change of one fully differentiated cell type to another.

Can you give an example?
In Barrett's oesophagus the distal stratified squamous epithelium is replaced by columnar epithelium like that present in the proximal stomach.

What mechanism is thought to be responsible?

Prolonged gastro-oesophageal reflux leads to inflammation and eventually ulceration. Healing occurs by re-epithelialisation, which in the acidic environment created by gastro-oesophageal reflux disease (GORD) differentiate into gastric or intestinal type epithelium. These are more resistant to injury from gastric contents.

How can Barrett's oesophagus be recognised macroscopically?

The gastro-oesophageal junction or Z-line moves proximally however this can be confused by the presence of a hiatus hernia. Barrett's oesophagus can be distinguished from stomach, as it is smooth and red while the stomach mucosa has longitudinal folds and has a more brownish colour.

What are the complications of Barrett's oesophagus?

- Ulceration, which can bleed, or stricture.
- Adenocarcinoma of the oesophagus.

3. Dysplasia

Define dysplasia.

Disorderly but non-neoplastic proliferation. The tissue shows cellular pleomorphism and loss of normal architecture but is not able to invade surrounding tissue.

Define carcinoma *in situ*.

Severe dysplasia is where the changes are severe and affect the whole thickness of epithelium so it has microscopic characteristics of malignancy but no evidence of invasion.

Give some causes of dysplasia.

- Smoking (bronchus).
- Alcohol (larynx).
- Chronic inflammation (bladder).
- Viral infection (cervix).

Describe some of the microscopic features seen in dysplasia.

- Cellular pleomorphism (variation in size/shape).
- Hyperchromatic nuclei.
- Increased number of mitoses.
- Abnormal position of mitoses (not confined to basal layer).

- Abnormal looking mitoses.
- Loss of cell–cell cohesion.
- Loss of normal architecture.

Which screening programmes are you aware of which aim to detect and monitor dysplasia?

- Cervical smears.
- Endoscopy for Barrett's oesophagus.
- Colonoscopy in longstanding ulcerative colitis.

DEATH, DAMAGE AND DEGENERATION

4. Ischaemia, Infarction and Necrosis

Define ischaemia and infarction.
- Ischaemia is an abnormal reduction in the blood supply or drainage of a tissue.
- Infarction is necrosis resulting from ischaemia.

What are the causes of ischaemia?
Ischaemia results from cellular anoxia or hypoxia, which in turn result from a variety of mechanisms including:

- Obstruction of arterial blood flow.
- Anaemia, a reduction in the number of oxygen-carrying red blood cells.
- Carbon monoxide poisoning, which reduces the oxygen-carrying capacity of red blood cells.
- Decreased perfusion of tissues by oxygen-carrying blood.
- Poor oxygenation of blood, secondary to pulmonary diseases.

What are the stages of ischaemic cell injury?
There are early and late stages of ischaemic cell injury. The early stage affects mitochondria, with the following consequences:

- Decreased oxidative phosphorylation and adenosine triphosphate (ATP) synthesis.
- Failure of the cell membrane Na^+/K^+ ATPase.
- Cellular swelling.
- Swelling of the endoplasmic reticulum.
- Swelling of the mitochondria.
- Disaggregation of ribosomes and failure of protein synthesis.
- Stimulation of phosphofructokinase activity.

The late stage of ischaemic cell injury results in membrane damage. This results in calcium influx into the cell, and cell death.

Are all cells as vulnerable to ischaemic injury?
No, vulnerability varies with tissue and cell type. Ischaemic injury becomes irreversible after: 3–5 minutes for neurones (Purkinje cells of the cerebellum, and the hippocampus are more susceptible than other neurones); 1–2 hours for cardiac myocytes and hepatocytes; >3 hours for skeletal muscle cells.

Define necrosis.
Necrosis is the abnormal death of individual cells within a living organism.

How do you classify necrosis?

- Coagulation necrosis: results from interruption of blood supply and there is preservation of tissue architecture; seen in organs supplied by end arteries, such as the heart and kidney.
- Liquefaction necrosis: enzymatic digestion of tissue; occurs with ischaemic injury to the central nervous system and from suppurative infections.
- Caseous necrosis: shows features of coagulation and liquefaction; occurs as part of granulomatous inflammation.
- Fat necrosis: traumatic or enzymatic (as in acute haemorrhagic pancreatitis).

What is the difference between wet and dry gangrene?

Dry gangrene is characterised primarily by coagulation necrosis without liquefaction. In wet gangrene the coagulation necrosis is complicated by infective heterolysis and consequent liquefaction necrosis.

What do you mean by heterolysis?

Heterolysis refers to cellular degradation by enzymes derived from extrinsic sources to the cell (e.g. bacteria). Autolysis refers to degradation caused by intracellular enzymes. Post-mortem autolysis occurs after death of the entire organism and so is not necrosis.

5. Atrophy, Aplasia, Agenesis and Apoptosis

Define atrophy.

Atrophy is a decrease in the size of an organ or tissue as a result of a decrease in mass of pre-existing cells. It most often results from disuse, nutritional or oxygen lack, diminished endocrine stimulation, ageing and denervation.

Define aplasia.

Aplasia is a failure of cell production. It follows the permanent loss of precursor cells in proliferative tissues.

Define agenesis.

During foetal development, aplasia results is agenesis, the absence of an organ due to failure of production.

What is apoptosis?

Apoptosis is the death of single cells within clusters of other cells.

Give some examples of where apoptosis occurs.

Apoptosis occurs as a physiological process for removal of cells during embryogenesis, during the endometrial cycle leading to menstruation, and as a pathological process as in the formation of Councilman bodies in viral hepatitis.

Do you know of any genes involved in apoptosis?

P53, *c-myc* and *Bcl-2*.

6. Wound Healing

List the factors associated with poor wound healing.

Local factors

- Poor blood supply (arterial deficiency, microvascular pathology or venous congestion).
- Infection.
- Haematoma.
- Local foreign material prejudicing healing, e.g. granulation tissue will not cover exposed subcutaneous metalwork.
- Previous radiotherapy injury.
- Local malignant metaplasia in chronic wounds.
- Exclude fistula or sinus formation.

Systemic factors

- Vitamin and trace element deficiency (vitamin C, zinc).
- Malnutrition.
- Drugs: immunosuppressants, cytotoxic agents, steroids and anticoagulants.
- Co-existent systemic disease, diabetes mellitus, anaemia, uraemia, jaundice/liver disease and malignancy.

What are the six phases of wound healing?

1. Haemostatic phase (platelet predominant).
2. Inflammatory phase 1 (neutrophil predominant).
3. Inflammatory phase 2 (macrophage predominant).
4. Proliferative phase/granulation tissue phase (fibroblast predominant, with neovascularisation).
5. Epithelialisation phase.
6. Remodelling phase.

Are the phases of wound healing discrete?

No. There is considerable overlap in the types and degree of cellular recruitment throughout wound healing. It is convenient to divide the phases up to commit to memory, but the cytokine cascade that conducts wound healing continually changes to involve the necessary players, as required.

What is the role of the macrophage in wound healing?

Macrophages have three principal roles:

1. Phagocytosis: clearing the debris of the initial inflammatory exudate and participating in extracellular matrix and collagen remodelling.

2. Bactericidal: killing of bacteria.
3. Production of various inflammatory mediators: cytokines, transforming growth factor B, monocyte chemotactic protein-1, fibroblast growth factor and vascular endothelial growth factor.

What is healing by primary intention?

In this situation the wound edges are closely opposed (e.g. a surgical incision closed by suturing). Healing requires minimal epidermal proliferation/formation of granulation tissue.

What is healing by secondary intention?

In this case a defect exists which is filled by formation of granulation tissue.

7. Organisation and Granulation

What does the term organisation refer to?

A fibrinous inflammatory exudate can form following tissue injury. If this cannot be removed by the body, it stimulates growth of fibroblasts and blood vessels (granulation tissue) with eventual conversion of the exudate into scar tissue. This process is known as organisation.

Which cells are responsible for removal of necrotic tissue during this process?

Phagocytic cells such as neutrophil polymorphs and macrophages.

Can you name a cytokine that stimulates ingress of these cells?

Transforming growth factor β.

Can you give an example of healing by organisation?

A fibrinous exudate fills the pleural cavity following acute lobar pneumonia. This cannot be completely removed but undergoes organisation, often leaving fibrous strands that bridge the pleural space.

What processes are involved in clearance of a venous thrombus by organisation?

This is a form of "intravascular" wound healing where the thrombus is organised into a scar within the vein. Initial stages involve an infiltration of macrophages which remove some of the thrombus. They may also orchestrate formation of small endothelial cell-lined channels within the thrombus which eventually coalesce and restore patency of the vein lumen. With time, a localised thickening of the vein wall may be the only remaining sign of thrombosis.

8. Fracture Healing

What are the immediate events that take place at the site of a bony fracture?

Haemorrhage within and around the bone results in formation of haematoma which will later provide a lattice for ingress and proliferation of cells. The devitalised fragments of soft tissue and bone are removed by neutrophils and macrophages.

What is the name given to new bone laid down following a fracture?

Callus.

Which cell is responsible for laying down callus and what is the pattern of deposition?

Callus is a mass of new bone laid down in an irregular, woven pattern by the osteoblast.

What is the fate of this callus?

It is eventually resorbed and replaced by lamellar bone which is laid in a more orderly fashion.

What are the factors that can delay fracture healing?

Systemic
- Poor circulation.
- Malnutrition.
- Systemic disease (e.g. malignancy).
- Drugs (corticosteroids, alcohol, smoking).

Local
- Movement of bone.
- Soft tissue interposition.
- Misalignment/distraction of bones.
- Infection.
- Malignancy.

9. Deposition and Stones

What types of renal tract calculi do you know?

- Calcium oxalate.
- Calcium phosphate.
- Magnesium ammonium phosphate.
- Urate.
- Cystine.

- Xanthine.
- Pyruvate.

What proportion of renal tract stones show up on plain radiographs?

The proportion is 90% (compared to only 10% of gallstones).

In what conditions do magnesium ammonium sulphate stones develop?

Alkaline urine, especially in the presence of *Proteus* infection, which can split urea molecules into ammonium. These stones are smooth and can enlarge rapidly hence they can fill the whole renal calyx, as is the case in stag-horn calculus.

What other factors can predispose to calculus formation?

- Dehydration.
- Urinary stasis.
- Infection.
- Hyperparathyroidism.
- Chemotherapy.
- Gout.
- Inherited metabolic abnormalities.

By what mechanism does a stone blocking the ureter lead to pain?

Backpressure of urine on the kidney stretches the renal capsule causing the classical severe constant pain. Spasm of the ureter is not thought to be the major cause of ureteric colic.

10. Acute Inflammation

What is acute inflammation?
This refers to the initial tissue reaction to an injurious agent.

What are the clinical features?
- Rubor (redness).
- Calor (heat).
- Tumor (swelling).
- Dolor (pain).
- Functio laesa (loss of function).

Do you know the main processes involved in an acute inflammatory response?
- Changes in vascular calibre.
- Increased vascular permeability.
- Formation of cellular exudate.
- Chemotaxis of neutrophils.
- Resolution.

How is the cellular exudate formed?
- Margination of neutrophils.
- Neutrophil adhesion to the vascular endothelium.
- Transmigration of leucocytes.
- Diapedesis.

What chemical mediators are involved in acute inflammation?
- Mediators producing changes in vascular calibre: histamine, complements (C5a and C3a) and prostaglandins.
- Mediators producing changes in vascular permeability: histamine and kinins.
- Mediators involved in chemotaxis: complement (C5a) and leucotrienes.

What are the possible sequelae of acute inflammation?
- Resolution: restoration of tissues to normal.
- Suppuration: pus formation due to excessive exudate.
- Repair and organisation: normal tissue is replaced by granulation tissue, as a result of excessive necrosis.
- Chronic inflammation: due to the persistence of a causal agent.

11. Chronic Inflammation

What is chronic inflammation?

Chronic inflammation refers to inflammation of prolonged duration. It may follow persistent infection, prolonged exposure to a toxic agent, repeated bouts of acute inflammation or be secondary to an auto-immune process.

What are the histological features of chronic inflammation?

- Infiltration of macrophages, lymphocytes and plasma cells.
- Tissue destruction.
- Fibrosis.

What is the role of macrophages in chronic inflammation?

In chronic inflammation, macrophages accumulate by the continued recruitment of monocytes, local proliferation of macrophages and immobilisation at the site by the action of cytokines. Macrophages release a number of substances that are either toxic to cells, lead to the influx of other cells and lead to proliferation of fibroblasts.

What are the features of a granulomatous inflammation?

This is a chronic inflammatory reaction characterised by the presence of epithelioid macrophages (granulomas) surrounded by a rim of lymphocytes.

Can you give any examples of conditions characterised by a granulomatous inflammation?

- Tuberculosis.
- Sarcoidosis.
- Brucellosis.
- Syphilis.
- Leprosy.

12. Inflammatory Cells

What are the main cells involved in acute inflammation?

- Neutrophil polymorphs.
- Mast cells.

What are the main cells involved in chronic inflammation?

- Macrophages.
- Lymphocytes.
- Plasma cells.

Mast cells and eosinophils are also present.

What are the functions of neutrophil polymorphs?

- Migration and chemotaxis.
- Phagocytosis.

How does phagocytosis occur?

Recognition and attachment by the phagocytic cell of particle to be ingested. This occurs only after the organism has been opsonised. The particle is then engulfed and degraded. Degradation can be through oxygen-dependent or oxygen-independent mechanisms. The main oxygen-dependent mechanism is the respiratory burst.

What are macrophages and how are they formed?

Macrophages are the main cell of chronic inflammation. They are a component of the mononuclear phagocyte system. Precursor cells in the bone marrow give rise to monocytes in the blood. These are converted to macrophages in tissues. They can either be activated to form cells such as giant cells and epitheloid cells or differentiate into tissue specific macrophages. They form microglia in the central nervous system (CNS), Kuppfer cells in the liver and alveolar macrophages in the lung.

What are the main functions of macrophages?

- Migration.
- Phagocytosis.
- Digestion.
- Formation of multi-nucleate giant cells.

13. Inflammatory Mediators

Do you know any chemical mediators of inflammation?

Inflammatory mediators can be derived from the plasma or from cells.

Plasma-derived mediators
- Complement system.
- Kinin system.
- Clotting system.
- Fibrinolytic system.

Cell-derived mediators

- Cytokines.
- Vasoactive amines.
- Arachidonic acid products.
- Lysosomal products.

What are the overall effects of these mediators?

- Vasodilatation.
- Increased vascular permeability.
- Emigration of neutrophils.
- Chemotaxis.
- Tissue damage.

Can you give any examples of vasoactive amines and how they act?

Histamine is released by mast cells and mediates the early phase of acute inflammation. Histamine causes vasodilatation and increase vascular permeability. Serotonin, released by platelets, is a potent vasoconstrictor.

What products of arachidonic acid are involved?

These are the prostaglandins and leucotrienes. Prostaglandins cause vasodilatation and increase vascular permeability. Leucotrienes also have vasoactive properties and increase vessel permeability.

What are cytokines? Can you give any examples?

These are small molecular weight peptides released from cells that influence the action of other cells through cell surface receptors. An important cytokine in inflammation is interleukin-8 (IL-8). This activates neutrophil polymorphs and promotes chemotaxis.

How is bradykinin produced and what is its role in inflammation?

Bradykinin is a product of the kinin system. Activated coagulation factor XII activates the conversion of prekallikrein to kallikrein. This in turn stimulates the conversion of kininogens to kinins such as bradykinin. Bradykinin acts as a vasodilator and increases vascular permeability. It is also a mediator of pain.

14. Tracts and Cavities

What is a sinus?

A sinus is a blind-ending tract lined by granulation tissue that communicates with an epithelial surface.

What is a fistula?

A fistula is an abnormal connection between two epithelialised surfaces.

Do you know any causes of fistulas?

- Direct injury.
- Infection.
- Persistent inflammation (e.g. Crohn's disease).
- Congenital fistulae.

What factors affect healing of sinuses or fistulas?

This can be divided into patient factors and local factors. Patient factors include malnutrition, vitamin deficiency, diabetes mellitus and immunosuppression. Local factors include infection, persistence of the causative agent, ischaemia and the presence of foreign material.

Can you give any examples of fistulas?

- Enterocutaneous fistula in Crohn's disease.
- Fistula in ano.

15. Innate Immunity

What are the features of innate immunity?

The innate immune system is the first-line defence to invading organisms. It is non-specific, non-adaptable, has no immunological memory and is present for life.

What are the components of the innate immune system?

- Physical barriers: skin, mucosa, secretions and cilia.
- Humoral: cytokines, soluble enzyme cascades (e.g. complement system) and opsonins (e.g. C-reactive protein).
- Cellular: neutrophils, monocytes/macrophages and natural killer cells.

What is complement?

Complement refers to a group of serum proteins produced in the liver that aid the action of antibody in the destruction of organisms. The complement system is a protein cascade containing more than 20 proteins. The complement proteins are soluble, though some are membrane bound. They are initially inactive and need to be sequentially activated for the cascade to proceed.

Do you know how the complement cascade works?

There are three pathways in the complement cascade: the alternative pathway (part of innate immunity), the classical pathway (part of specific immune system) and the common pathway.

- The classical pathway is activated by antibody–antigen complexes. The formation of the immune complex induces a conformational change in the structure that allows it to bind to complement component C1. C4 and C2 combine to form C4b2a (classical pathway C3 convertase). This catalyses the conversion of C3 to C3b and combines with C3b to form C5 convertase, which cleaves C5, a component of the common pathway.
- The alternative pathway is activated by a bacterium. C3b is required for activation of the pathway. C3b from the classical pathway combines with factors B and D to form the alternative pathway C3 convertase. This combines with C3b to form the alternative pathway C5 convertase initiating the common pathway.
- The common pathway involves the sequential activation of complement proteins leading to the formation of the membrane attack complex which acts as the killer molecule. This inserts into the cell membrane and causes cell death by osmotic lysis.

What are the effects of complement activation?

- Bacterial cell lysis.
- Solubilisation of antibody–antigen complexes.
- Activation of mast cells and basophils.
- Recruitment of neutrophils.

16. Specific Immunity

What are the features of specific immunity?

- Specificity.
- Immunological memory.
- Variable intensity of response.
- Recognition of self and non-self.

What are the components of the adaptive immune system?

- Cellular: mediated by T and B lymphocytes.
- Humoral: mediated by antibodies or cytokines.

What are the functions of B lymphocytes?

- Formation of antibodies and lymphokines.
- Activation of T cells, macrophages and plasma cells.

- Chemotaxis.
- Cell lysis.

What are the functions of T lymphocytes?

T cells are involved in cell-mediated immunity. They recognise antigen on the surface of major histocompatibility complex (MHC) cells. CD4 cells recognise antigen fragments on MHC class II cells and aid production of antibodies by B cells. CD8 cells recognise antigen fragments on MHC class I cells. They are cytotoxic for intracellular pathogens.

How are immunoglobulins subdivided?

There are five classes of immunoglobulin (Ig):

- IgA: dimeric.
- IgG: monomeric.
- IgD: monomeric.
- IgE: monomeric.
- IgM: pentameric.

What is the difference between a primary and secondary antibody response?

When an antigen is encountered for the first time, an antibody response can be detected after 5–10 days. This response rises slowly over the next 2 weeks before declining to a low level. The primary response involves mainly IgM class antibody.

If the same antigen is encountered again, there is a more rapid antibody response, with a higher peak level of antibody. This secondary response is mediated predominantly by IgG. It is antigen specific, has acquired memory and is of higher intensity to the primary response.

17. Immunodeficiency

How can you classify immunodeficiency?

Immunodeficiency can be classified as either primary (inherited) or secondary (acquired). It can also be classified on the basis of the immune component affected:

- T cell deficiency.
- B cell deficiency.
- Combined B and T cell deficiency.
- Neutrophil defects.
- Deficiency of complement components.

Can you give any examples of each one?

- T cell deficiency: Di George syndrome and acquired immunodeficiency syndrome (AIDS).

- B cell deficiency: X-linked agammaglobulinaemia and selective IgA deficiency.
- Combined B and T cell deficiency: severe combined immunodeficiency and Wiskott–Aldrich syndrome.
- Neutrophil defects: chronic granulomatous disease and leukocyte adhesion deficiency.
- Complement deficiency: any non-specific classical pathway deficiency.

What are the main causes of secondary immunodeficiency?

- Age.
- Malnutrition.
- Neoplasia, e.g. lymphoma.
- Infection (AIDS).
- Drugs (corticosteroids and immunosuppressants).
- Connective tissue disorders.

Why does a splenectomy lead to immunological impairment?

The spleen carries out a number of immunological functions. It is a major site of antibody production and possesses a reservoir of lymphocytes. In addition, it is a site for the phagocytosis of opsonised bacteria and parasites. Splenectomy leads to an impaired antibody response with increased susceptibility to infection.

How does the stress of surgery lead to immunodeficiency?

- Breach of mucosal and epithelial barriers.
- Decreased production of interferons after trauma.
- Depletion of complement in hypercatabolic states.
- Fall in antibody production.
- Phagocyte dysfunction.

18. Hypersensitivity

What do you understand by the term "hypersensitivity reaction"?

This describes a series of reactions where contact with antigen induces an exaggerated immune response resulting in tissue damage. These are initiated by antibody–antigen interactions or cell-mediated mechanisms.

How would you classify hypersensitivity reactions?

Hypersensitivity reactions are classified on by the immunological mechanism that mediates the disease. They are classified as type I to type IV reactions.

What is type I hypersensitivity?

This is a rapidly developing immune reaction. Antigen combines with IgE antibodies bound to mast cells in a previously sensitised individual. This leads to mast cell degranulation with release of histamine and other mediators of inflammation.

Examples include asthma, eczema, allergic rhinitis, urticaria and generalised anaphylaxis.

What is anaphylaxis?

Anaphylaxis is the clinical manifestation of a generalised IgE-mediated immune reaction. The allergen must be systemically absorbed for the reaction to occur. A patient may present with widespread urticaria and angio-oedema. Serious sequelae include bronchial spasm, laryngeal oedema and death.

What is type II hypersensitivity?

Antibodies (which are not IgE) interact with antigen on the surface of cells. Complement is activated leading to cell death and mast cell activation.

Can you give some examples of type II hypersensitivity?

- Autoimmune diseases, e.g. myaesthenia gravis and glomerulonephritis.
- Pernicious anaemia.
- Transfusion reactions.
- Hyperacute allograft rejection.

What is type III hypersensitivity?

Type III differs from type II in that circulating immune complexes are formed. Antibody–antigen complexes are either deposited in tissues or form within tissues (the latter is the Arthus reaction). Complement is activated leading to tissue damage.

Can you give some examples of type II hypersensitivity?

- Extrinsic allergic alveolitis.
- Post-streptococcal nephritis.
- Subacute bacterial endocarditis.
- Polyarteritis nodosa.

What is type IV hypersensitivity?

This is a cell-mediated reaction, initiated by sensitised T lympho-cytes. CD4 T cells initiate delayed hypersensitivity reactions. CD8 T cells mediate direct cell toxicity.

Can you give some examples of type II hypersensitivity?

- Tuberculosis: the immunological reaction to *Mycobacterium tuberculosis* leads to granuloma formation.
- Contact dermatitis, e.g. nickel allergy.

19. Tumour Nomenclature and Definitions

What do you understand by the term neoplasia?

Neoplasia was defined by Willis as an abnormal mass of tissue, the growth of which:

1. is uncoordinated,
2. exceeds that of normal tissues,
3. persists in the same manner after the cessation of the stimulus which (presumably) evoked the change.

What is the difference between a benign and a malignant neoplasm and why is this distinction important?

The distinction as to whether a neoplasm is benign or malignant is crucial in understanding the natural history of the neoplasm and in the selection of the most appropriate treatment. Ultimately, the distinction between benign and malignant is a behavioural one and there are certain morphological and structural features that correlate with these patterns of behaviour. In morphological terms, benign tumours show a normal arrangement of tissue cells and have an expansile growth pattern, whereas malignant tumours tend to show disrupted intercellular relationships and an infiltrative growth pattern. There are also more nuclear abnormalities seen in malignant tumours. In structural terms, benign tumours tend to be polypoid or papillary, whereas malignant tumours are more likely to be fungating, ulcerating or annular lesions.

How else are neoplasms classified?

Neoplasms can be classified according to whether they are epithelial or stromal.

How are benign epithelial neoplasms named?

Epithelial neoplasms are named according to the type of epithelium (squamous, transitional and columnar) from which they are derived their morphological features: adenoma (glandular pattern or deriving from a gland), papilloma (protruding from surface) or cystadenoma (lumen of a gland blocked by tumour thereby causing glandular distension). For example, squamous cell papilloma or transitional cell adenoma.

How are benign stromal neoplasms named?

By adding the suffix -oma to the tissue of origin, e.g. fibroma, osteoma and haemangioma.

What is the difference between a sarcoma and a carcinoma?

Malignant tumours of epithelial composition are known as carcinomas and malignant tumours of mesenchymal composition are known as sarcomas. It is important to appreciate that it is the cellular composition of the tumour that determines whether it is a carcinoma or sarcoma and not the germ cell of origin.

What is the difference between tumour grading and tumour staging and why are these useful tools?

Grading is the process by which characteristic histological features, e.g. degree of mitotic activity and nuclear size, are used to assess the aggressive potential of a tumour. Grading is most important in situations where complete removal of a tumour may not be possible for technical reasons, i.e. grading assists in making a decision as to whether or not to operate on a tumour which is difficult to excise. Staging, on the other hand, is more relevant in making decisions in tumours that are technically more feasible to resect. Staging refers to the size and spread of a tumour.

Can you give one example of tumour grading and tumour staging systems?

- Gleason's grading for prostate cancer.
- Tumour necrosis metastasis (TNM) staging for breast cancer (also Duke's for colonic cancer).

20. Carcinogenesis

How would you categorise factors that are implicated in carcinogenesis?

The factors implicated in carcinogenesis can be broadly divided into genetic and environmental (chemical carcinogens and radiation).

What types of genes do you know that have been implicated in carcinogenesis?

Oncogenes, tumour suppressor genes and apoptosis regulatory genes.

What are oncongenes and can you give some examples?

Oncogenes are genes that can lead to the formation of malignant cells if their gene product is altered or abnormally expressed. Oncogenes are transformed from proto-oncogenes by mutations, chromosomal rearrangements or gene amplification. Three well-known oncogenes are:

- *Ras*: Encodes a G-protein and if mutated the G-protein remains in its growth-activating state. Implicated in colonic, lung, pancreatic cancer and melanomas.
- *Myc*: A transcriptional activator whose activity is increased by either translocation (Burkitt's lymphoma) or gene amplification (some small cell carcinomas).
- *HER2*: HER2 also encodes for a protein homologue of tyrosine kinase growth factor receptors and its amplification is associated with aggressive behaviour in certain breast tumours.

What are tumour suppressor genes and can you give an example?

Tumour suppressor genes encode proteins that prevent or retard tumour cell proliferation. If their function is disrupted tumours are more likely to occur. The p53 is the commonest gene to be altered in human cancers (it is found in 70% of colon cancers and over one-third of breast cancers).

What is the classical evidence for the role of tumour suppressor genes in cell proliferation?

- Hybrid cell studies: fusion of malignant and normal cells suppresses tumour formation.
- Hereditary tumours: alteration of certain genes associated with hereditary cancers.
- Transfection studies: transfection of wild-type suppressor genes into tumour cells may restore the non-tumourigenic phenotype.

What is Knudson's "two-hit" hypothesis?

Knudson's 'two-hit' hypothesis is that both alleles of a tumour suppressor gene must be damaged or deleted for transformation to the tumourigenic phenotype to occur. This was based on observations in hereditary and non-hereditary retinoblastomas.

21. Natural History of Malignancy

What is the cell cycle?

The cell cycle refers to the different stages a cell goes through in order to divide.

What are the different stages of the cell cycle?

- G1 phase (Gap 1): mitosis has just been completed, this is a presynthetic stage of unknown processes.

- S phase (synthesis phase): synthesis of cellular components.
- G2 phase (Gap 2): premitotic phase with no obvious events related to cell division.
- M phase: mitotic phase.
- G0 phase: a resting phase that some cells will enter before moving onto G1 phase again.

What is the significance of the cell cycle to malignant tumour growth?

In the adult cell, division continues (except for the central nervous system) without an increase in the total number of cells; there are complex processes controlling cell division. In tumour cells, this control appears to be lost and cell division increases the population of tumour cells. It is important to realise, however, that cell division of tumours is not necessarily disorganised and the cell cycle of a tumour cell may closely resemble that of a normal cell.

What controls the doubling time of a tumour?

- The number of cells dividing.
- The rate of division.
- The rate of cell loss.

Are there any differences between tumour types?

Yes, leucaemias show exponential growth whereas solid tumours grow much more slowly. For example, a solid tumour in the breast may double over 30 times before it becomes palpable clinically.

What do you understand by the clonal evolution?

The concept of clonal evolution is that a genetic mutation in a single cell can cause replication of cells in unusual circumstances. Some of the daughter cells will undergo further mutations and there will be further loss of control of cell division. Eventually, a population of cells will exist that show the malignant phenotype.

What is the significance of angiogenesis to tumour growth?

Angiogenesis is required in order for a solid tumour to keep expanding in size. Angiogenesis may also increase the risk of metastasis of a tumour.

What do you understand by the term 'natural history' in relation to tumours?

This term is used to describe what will happen to a tumour if left to run its natural course. This will differ for different types of tumour.

For example, some tumours will have metastasised by the time they present clinically. Other tumours are extremely indolent and may not be a threat to life for many years. Different tumours also have different patterns of metastasis, e.g. bronchial carcinoma metastases to bone, brain, liver and adrenal glands, whereas renal carcinoma metastasises primarily to the lung.

22. Cancer Screening

How can screening be defined?
Any medical test that does not arise from a patient's request for advice about a specific condition.

Can you name some tumours that are screened for in the UK?
- Breast cancer.
- Colorectal cancer: only in selected individuals, e.g. patients with familial adenomatous polyposis.

Is this same in other countries?
No. In Japan there is screening for gastric cancer which has a greater incidence there than in the UK.

What is meant by the lag time bias of a screening test?
Since a screening test identifies disease before it has presented clinically it will appear to increase survival measured from the time of diagnosis. For example, a patient presents with a malignant breast tumour and survives 30 years. If the tumour had been identified a year earlier by screening then the survival since diagnoses would have been 31 years.

What are the potential advantages of screening for cancers?
- Improved prognosis.
- Treatment regimes may be less radical for disease found at an earlier stage.
- Reassurance of patients without pathology.

What are the potential disadvantages of screening for cancers?
- Treatment may not always alter outcome, therefore morbidity will be longer due to early diagnosis.
- Screening test may be invasive and have associated complications.
- False positives may lead to unnecessary treatment.

23. Management of Maligancy

What are the overall goals in managing malignancy?

- To achieve local control of the tumour.
- To prevent/treat metastases.
- To improve quality of life.
- To alleviate pain and psychological distress.

If an operation is available, should all primary tumours be operated upon?

No, there are many reasons that would make it inappropriate to operate on a primary tumour, e.g. the operation is unlikely to improve survival, or there may be other less invasive forms of treatment available.

If an operation will not improve long-term survival, are there any other reasons to perform the operation?

An operation may be performed for palliative reasons to relieve pain.

A patient is referred to a neurosurgical unit with a brain tumour that appears to be inoperable. Why might a biopsy be offered to the patient?

To obtain a histological diagnosis and plan adjuvant therapy such as radiotherapy and chemotherapy.

What other information about a tumour is useful in planning the treatment regime?

The stage of the tumour, e.g. the TNM stage (takes into account tumour grade, nodal status and metastases).

24. Components of Blood

What are the constituents of blood?
Blood is made up of plasma, within which are suspended erythrocytes, leucocytes and platelets.

What is contained in plasma?
The majority of plasma is water (approximately 95%). In addition, it contains ions – the principal cation is sodium, with chloride as the principal anion. Other ions such as K^+, Mg^{2+}, Ca^{2+} and HCO_3^- are present in smaller quantities. Other constituents of plasma include glucose, fatty acids, cholesterol and the plasma proteins – albumins, globulins and fibrinogen.

What are the different types of leucocyte?
They can be subdivided into the granulocytes and agranulocytes. Granulocytes contain segmented nuclei. The granulocytes can be further divided into neutrophils, eosinophils and basophils according to their staining characteristics. The agranulocytes can be further divided into monocytes and lymphocytes.

What are the functions of erythrocytes?
The main function of red cells is to transport oxygen and carbon dioxide. They are small biconcave cells that have a large surface area to allow efficient gas exchange. The erythrocyte contains the oxygen-binding protein haemoglobin.

How are blood cells formed?
Blood cells are formed by haematopoiesis. All cells are formed from pluripotent stem cells. This precursor cell gives rise to lymphoid stem cells and myeloid stem cells. The lymphoid stem cells migrate to lymphoid organs and are responsible for differentiating into B and T lymphocytes. Myeloid stem cells remain in the bone marrow and differentiate into colony-forming cells that produce erythrocytes, platelets, granulocytes and monocytes.

Can you briefly outline erythropoiesis?
Erythroblasts are the precursor cell to erythrocytes. Erythropoietin regulates the differentiation of stem cells into erythroblasts. Through a series of cell divisions, erythroblasts differentiate into reticulocytes in the bone marrow. Reticulocytes mature into erythrocytes in peripheral blood.

25. Haemostasis I: Clots, Thrombus and Coagulation

What is a clot?

A clot is a mass of material that is formed from the coagulation of stationary blood.

How does this differ from a thrombus?

A thrombus is a mass of material formed from the coagulation of blood in either a blood vessel or the heart.

What are the components of a normal haemostatic response?

The normal homoeostatic response depends on the coordinated interactions between the vessel wall, platelets and coagulation pathways.

What is the role of platelets?

The main function is the formation of a mechanical plug. This is achieved by:

1. Platelet adhesion to exposed endothelial connective tissue through the action of von Willebrand factor.
2. Secretion of platelet granule contents including adenosine diphosphate (ADP), serotonin, thromboxanes and prostaglandins.
3. Platelet aggregation under control of ADP and thromboxane A_2.
4. Release of platelet-derived growth factor, which aids vascular healing after injury.

Can you describe the coagulation cascade?

The coagulation cascade involves the sequential activation of clotting factors that eventually leads to fibrin formation. Three pathways are involved: an intrinsic pathway, an extrinsic pathway and final common pathway. The intrinsic pathway is dependent on contact factors which activates factor XII. This in turn leads to the sequential activation of factors XI, IX and X. The extrinsic pathway is tissue factor dependent. This activates factor VII, which in turn activates factor X. In the final common pathway, activated factor X converts prothrombin to thrombin. Thrombin converts fibrinogen to fibrin in the formation of a fibrin clot.

Can you give any causes of abnormal bleeding?

*   Vascular bleeding disorders, e.g. vascular purpuras.
*   Thrombocytopaenia.
*   Platelet function defects.
*   Disorders of coagulation.

Do you know any examples of disorders of coagulation?

Congenital
- Haemophilia A.
- Factor IX deficiency.
- Von Willebrand's disease.

Acquired
- Vitamin K deficiency.
- Liver disease.
- Disseminated intravascular coagulation (DIC).

What is DIC?

The intravascular deposition of fibrin with the associated consumption of platelets and coagulation factors.

Can you tell me some causes of DIC?

- Infection (especially Gram-negative septicaemia).
- Malignancy.
- Anaphylaxis.
- Post-surgery or trauma.
- Shock.
- Burns.
- Hypothermia.
- Amniotic fluid embolism.

26. Haemostasis II: Bleeding and Thrombotic Disorders

What factors predispose to thrombosis?

Virchow's triad: alterations in normal blood flow, endothelial wall damage and hypercoagulability. Arterial thrombosis is more strongly associated with intimal damage of the endothelial wall. Venous thrombosis is associated more with stasis and hypercoagulability.

What factors affect altered blood flow?

- Turbulent flow: prosthetic heart valves and atherosclerotic stenosis.
- Stasis: aneurysms, prolonged immobility, cardiac failure, pelvic obstruction and dehydration.

Can you give any causes of endothelial wall damage?

- Atherosclerosis.
- Intravenous cannulae.

- Smoking.
- Bacterial endotoxins.
- Vasculitis.

Can you give any examples of a hypercoagulable state?
Congenital
- Protein C and S deficiency.
- Anti-thrombin III deficiency.
- Factor V Leiden gene mutation.

Acquired
- Oral contraceptive pill.
- Surgery.
- Malignancy.
- Pregnancy.

What is the fate of the thrombus?
The thrombus can undergo organisation, dissolution, propagation and embolisation.

What is an embolus?
A mass of undissolved material of solid, liquid or gaseous origin that is carried in the blood to a site distant from its origin.

Can you give some causes of embolism?
- Venous embolism: from thrombosis of deep leg veins.
- Arterial embolism: myocardial infarction and atrial fibrillation.
- Fat embolism.
- Gas embolism: gas entering the blood stream, e.g. during surgery, or gas dissolved in blood coming out of solution, e.g. nitrogen.
- Amniotic fluid embolism: occurs at placental membrane rupture with rupture of veins in uterine wall.
- Tumour embolism.
- Cholesterol embolism.
- Injection of foreign material.
- Therapeutic embolisation.

27. Anaemia

What is anaemia?
Anaemia is defined as a haemoglobin concentration of $<13.5\,\mathrm{g/dl}$ in adult males and $11.5\,\mathrm{g/dl}$ in adult females.

What are the physiological responses to anaemia?

Acutely, tachycardia and an increase in cardiac output. Oxygen extraction from blood is increased resulting in a lower PaO_2 in venous blood. Chronically, an increase in erythropoietin secretion by the kidneys.

How would you classify anaemia?

- Microcytic, hypochromic (mean corpuscular volume (MCV): <80 fl).
- Normochromic, normocytic (MCV: 80–95 fl).
- Macrocytic: megaloblastic or non megaloblastic (MCV: >95 fl).

Do you know any causes of a microcytic anaemia?

The commonest cause is iron deficiency anaemia. Other causes include thalassaemia, sideroblastic anaemia and anaemia of chronic disease.

What tests would you perform to differentiate an iron deficiency anaemia from anaemia of chronic disease?

In iron deficiency anaemia, the serum iron and ferritin are low. Serum transferrin is raised. The erythrocyte sedimentation rate (ESR) is elevated in proportion to the anaemia. The blood film reveals target cells and elliptocytes (pencil cells). In anaemia of chronic disease, serum iron and transferrin are low. Serum ferritin is raised. ESR is elevated out of proportion to the anaemia. The blood film shows marked rouleaux formation.

What are the causes of a normochromic, normocytic anaemia?

- Anaemia of chronic disease.
- Post-acute blood loss.
- Bone marrow failure.
- Haemolytic anaemia.
- Mixed deficiencies.

Do you know any causes of a macrocytic anaemia.

- Megaloblastic: B_{12} and folate deficiency.
- Non-megaloblastic: alcohol, liver disease, hypothyroidism, aplastic anaemias and myelodysplastic syndromes.

What would be your initial investigations of a macrocytic anaemia?

- Serum B_{12} and red cell folate.
- Liver function tests.
- Thyroid function tests.

- Reticulocyte count.
- Bone marrow aspirate.

What are the blood film features of a macrocytic anaemia?

- Megaloblastic anaemia: oval macrocytes with marked anisocytosis, tear-drop poikilocytes, and red cell fragments and hypersegmented neutrophils.
- Non-megaloblastic anaemia: round macrocytes without marked anisocytosis and poikilocytosis, and normal neutrophil segmentation.

28. Transfusion

What blood group systems do you know about?
The blood group systems that are most commonly in use are the ABO and the Rhesus system.

The ABO system consists of three allelic genes A, B and O producing four phenotypes, namely O, A, B, AB:

Phenotypes	Antigens	Antibodies
O	O	Anti-A and anti-B
A	A	Anti-B
B	B	Anti-A
AB	AB	None

Do you know what blood components are available for transfusion?
- Whole blood.
- Red cells: plasma reduced.
- Fresh frozen plasma (leucocyte depleted, frozen and phenotyped).
- Plasma products: albumin, coagulation factors and immunoglobulins
- Platelets.

Can you tell me some of the early side effects associated with blood transfusions?
Immunological
- Haemolytic transfusion reaction.
- Anaphylactic.
- Febrile non-haemolytic reaction.
- Transfusion-related acute lung injury.

Non-immunological
- Bacterial contamination.
- Endotoxins.
- Hypocalcaemia.
- Hyperkalaemia
- Fluid overload.
- Air embolism.
- Clotting abnormalities.

Do you know any delayed adverse effects of blood transfusions?

Immunological
- Delayed haemolytic transfusion reactions.
- Graft versus host disease.
- Post-transfusion purpura.

Non-immunological
- Infection.
- Transfusional iron overload.

What infections can be transmitted by transfusions?

- Bacterial: *Treponema pallidum* (syphilis), *Salmonella* and *Brucella*.
- Viral: hepatitis A, B, C; human immunodeficiency virus 1 and 2 (HIV-1 and HIV-2, respectively); parvovirus; cytomegalovirus; and Epstein–Barr virus.
- Protozoal: *Plasmodium* sp. (malaria); *Toxoplasma*; *Trypanosoma cruzi* (Chagas' disease).
- Prion: new variant Creutzfeldt–Jakob diseases (CJD).

Is there any alternative to help prevent adverse effects?

Yes, autologous blood transfusion. This can be achieved by re-operative donation, acute normovolaemic haemodilution (removal of blood prior to surgery with crystalloid replacement) or peri-operative red cell salvage.

MICROBIOLOGY

29. Classification of Microbes

What type of organism is a virus?
Viruses are obligate intracellular parasites relying on host cells for replication. They consist of a package of DNA or RNA within a protein coat.

How can viruses be subdivided into classes?
- By family, e.g. adenovirus and herpes virus.
- By genomic type, i.e. single- and double-stranded RNA or DNA.

Define and describe a protozoa.
Protozoa are single-celled organisms, which are motile, have a membrane and have complex organelles in their cytoplasm.

What are helminths?
Parasitic worms with complex life cycles. They are well-differentiated multi-cellular organisms.

What type of organism are bacteria?
Single-cell organisms lacking nuclei and endoplasmic reticulum but with a cell wall.

How do fungi differ from bacteria?
Fungi have a nucleus, are bigger and can reproduce sexually.

30. Spread of Infection

Describe some routes by which infection can spread.
- Droplet inhalation.
- Eating infected food.
- Sexual intercourse.
- Blood-borne infection and blood transfusion.
- Via insect bite.
- Faeco-oral transmission.
- Saliva.
- Transplacental spread from mother to foetus.

What reservoirs of infection can you name?
- People (including medical staff).
- Animals.

- Air.
- Soil.
- Food.
- Water.

What sort of infection has the capacity to spread widely?

One that is easily transmitted (e.g. droplet) and has a latent period before causing symptoms. Also non-mobile populations living in close proximity and with no herd immunity also help proliferation of the infection.

What recent disease outbreak exemplifies these characteristics?

SARS: severe acute respiratory syndrome.

What other difficulties did doctors face in dealing with SARS ?

- Not easy to diagnose.
- Hospital staff infected.

31. Defence Against Infection

What is the first barrier to infection of any micro-organism faces?

Intact skin and mucosa are a natural barrier to infection and breaks in the skin or mucosa are more vulnerable. The majority of skin infections occur secondary to damage, e.g. wounds or burns.

What mucosal secretions can you think of which act as a defence against micro-organisms?

- Stomach acid.
- Lysozymes from tear glands degrade bacterial cell walls and protect the eye.

What are the differences between the innate and the adaptive immune systems?

The innate immune system cannot respond to organisms, which have developed defences against it, does not respond to specific antigens and does not develop memory (increased response on second exposure to a pathogen).

What are the two arms of the adaptive immune system?

Cell-mediated immunity and humoural immunity (carried out by cytokines and antibodies).

How does antibody binding lead to killing of micro-organisms?

Antibody binding can activate the complement system, which in turn can opsonise bacteria (make them more easily phagocytosed) or kill them directly by forming the membrane attack complex. Antibody binding itself can opsonise organism by binding surface receptors with its Fc component.

Any individual has around 10^{10} different antibodies, how is such variation generated?

Antibodies are coded for by V (variability), D (diversity) and J (joining) genes for each of which multiple copies are inherited. Massive further variation occurs as the V genes have mutation hotspots in their hypervariable regions.

32. Bacteriology Basics

What are Koch's postulates?

The criteria for linking a micro-organism to a disease:

1. The organism can be isolated from lesions of the disease.
2. Inoculation of the organism causes a lesion in an animal model.
3. The organism can be removed from lesions in the animal model.

What is the Gram stain?

A staining technique using crystal violet and then a counterstain with safranin.

What colours do Gram-positive and Gram-negative bacteria appear?

- Gram-positives: blue-purple.
- Gram-negatives: pink-red.

What shapes of bacteria are commonly seen?

- Cocci: spheres, in chains or clumps.
- Bacilli: rods.
- Spirochetes: spirals.
- Vibrios: comma shaped.

Name a Gram-negative coccus.
Neisseria meningitides (or *Gonococcus*).

Name an anaerobic Gram-negative bacillus.
Pseudomonas.

33. *Staphylococcus* and *Streptococcus*

What category of bacteria are *Staphylococcus* and *Streptococcus*?
Gram-positive cocci.

How are the *streptococci* subdivided?
Broadly by the ability to haemolyse red blood cells in blood-containing medium – haemolytic:

- partial haemolysis,
- complete haemolysis,
- no haemolysis.

They are then further subdivided by serology based on surface poly-saccharide antigens into Lancefield groups.

To which antibiotic are *Streptococci* most sensitive?
Penicillin.

How are the *Staphylococci* subdivided?
- Coagulase positive, e.g. *Staphylococcus aureus*.
- Coagulase negative, e.g. *Staphylococcus epidermis*.

What infections have you seen caused by *Staphylococcus aureus*?
- Wound infections.
- Abscesses.
- Septicaemia.
- Pneumonia.
- Toxic shock syndrome.

Discuss the antibiotic sensitivity of *Staphylococcus aureus*.
It is increasingly antibiotic resistant. Although traditionally sensitive to β-lactams, methicillin-resistant *Staphylococcus aureus* (MRSA) is an increasing problem requiring treatment with vancomycin and teicoplanin.

34. Clostridia

What type of organism is clostridium?
Anaerobic Gram-positive bacillus (rod). *Clostridia* are spore forming and produce an exotoxin. They are saprophytic, i.e. they live in soil.

Which types of clostridia cause disease in man?
1. *Clostridium tetani*: tetanus.
2. *Clostridium difficile*: pseudomembranous colitis.
3. *Clostridium perfringens* (*welchii*): gas gangrene.
4. *Clostridium botulinum*: food poisoning.

Which patients are most at risk of pseudomembranous colitis?
Elderly patients treated with broad-spectrum antibiotics in hospital. The organism is spore bearing so survives well in the hospital environment.

Describe how the disease arises, presents and is diagnosed.
Clostridium difficile overgrows gut flora after antibiotic treatment. The *clostridia* release multiple toxins, which damage the membrane of epithelial cells causing ulceration and leading to the formation of a pseudomembrane. The patient develops fever and profuse diarrhoea. The pseudomembrane can be seen on sigmoidoscopy. *Clostridium difficile* can be cultured from stool specimens but this does not prove that it is responsible for symptoms; assays are used to demonstrate the presence of the toxin.

How is *Clostridium difficile* treated?
Supportive measures should be initiated and broad-spectrum antibiotics stopped. Vancomycin or metronidazole are usually started depending on local policy.

35. Tuberculosis

What type of micro-organism causes tuberculosis?
Tuberculosis results from infection by *Mycobacterium tuberculosus*, an aerobic, non-spore forming, non-motile bacillus with a waxy coat.

What diagnostic tests do you know of for tuberculosis?
Acid-fast stains such as Ziehl–Neelson stain the waxy coat if a smear contains a large number of organisms. Growth in culture allows

identification of the organism and study of drug sensitivities however mycobacteria grow 20–100 times more slowly than other bacteria so this can take 4–6 weeks. An injection of a pure protein derivative of *Mycobacterium tuberculosus* under the skin is known as the tuberculin test (or heaf test) and use delayed hypersensitivity. A positive test shows previous exposure but does not prove active infection. More rapid diagnosis is now possible using polymerase chain reaction (PCR) to amplify RNA.

What are the commonest sites of infection for primary tuberculosis?

- Lung.
- Tonsils.
- Terminal ileum.

Explain the natural history of untreated tuberculous adenitis.

The *Mycobacterium* enters through the tonsil and spread to the ipsilateral cervical lymph nodes. The nodes caseate and can liquefy and break down to form a cold abscess. The pus is initially trapped inside the deep cervical fascia. Over time a point in the fascia will erode to form a hole allowing the pus to pass into the space below the superficial fascia. This is the "collar-stud" abscess which left untreated will enlarge leading to skin reddening, formation of a fluctuant swelling and eventually rupture and sinus formation.

What are the principles of treating tuberculous adenitis?

The mainstay of treatment is anti-tuberculous drugs given as triple or quadruple therapy guided by the sensitivity of aspirated pus. If medical treatment fails to resolve the abscess excision of the fibrous capsule may be necessary although this can be technically challenging.

36. Anaerobes

What would make you think an infected wound had anaerobic bacteria involved?

Clinical suspicion from the mechanism but also the distinctive and terrible smell.

How can anaerobes be classified?

They can be divided into obligate and facultative anaerobes. Obligate anaerobes cannot grow in the presence of oxygen. They can also be divided into spore-formers, e.g. *clostridia*, and the non-spore-formers from the alimentary canal. Like all bacteria they can be categorised by their appearance on Gram stain:

- Gram-positive cocci: *peptostreptococci*.
- Gram-positive bacilli: *clostridia*.
- Gram-negative bacilli: *Bacteroides*.

Apart from not forming spores in what other ways do non-spore forming anaerobes differ from *clostridia*?

They are not toxin producing and they are opportunistic pathogens.

What are the commonest aetiologies of gas gangrene?

Trauma and bowel/gall bladder surgery.

How do gas bubbles develop?

Clostridium perfringens infection results in extensive oedema and muscle necrosis. Bacterial fermentation within the gangrenous tissues results in gas bubbles. Massive proteolysis from enzyme action cause further tissue necrosis.

37. Gut Organisms

Define endogenous and exogenous infection?

- Endogenous: infection by an organism normally found in the patient.
- Exogenous: infection acquired from an external source such as medical staff, equipment or other patients.

What is the normal flora of the lower gastro-intestinal (GI) tract?

- Gram-negative bacilli: *Escherichia coli*, *Klebsiella*.
- Gram-positive cocci: *Enterococcus faecalis*, *Pseudomonas*, *Enterobacter*.
- Anaerobes: *Bacteroides*.

This variety of flora contributes to the extensive risk of wound infection if the bowel contents are spilled.

What prophylactic antibiotics would you recommend for colorectal surgery?

It is necessary to cover anaerobes and Gram-negative rods, therefore a typical combination includes: metronidazole + second generation cephalosporin ± gentamicin.

What mechanisms do enteropathic bacteria use to cause GI tract disease?

- Release of enterotoxins, e.g. *Staphylococcus* food poisoning.
- Release of exotoxin causing gut epithelium to secrete excess volumes of fluid leading to watery diarrhoea, e.g.*Vibrio cholera*.
- Invasion of, and damage to, the epithelium causing ulceration and bleeding, e.g. *Shigella, Campylobacter*.
- Passage through the mucosa and mesenteric lymph nodes to enter blood, causing bacteraemia, e.g. *Salmonella*.

When might fungi invade the GI tract?

In an immunocompromised patient, e.g. *Candida* infecting the oesophagus as an acquired immunodeficiency syndrome (AIDS) defining illness.

38. Bacterial Toxins

What is an exotoxin?

A protein secreted from an organism that has a specific molecular target. They are immunogenic and damaged by heat.

What is an endotoxin?

A lipopolysaccharide (LPS) from the outer cell wall of Gram-negative bacteria. They are heat stable, non-immunogenic and have a broad spectrum of effect.

How does an endotoxin act?

LPS induces fever, macrophage activation and B lymphocyte activity via cytokine formation, e.g. tumour necrosis factor (TNF) and interleukin-1 (IL-1). These have broad effects, including:

- Prostaglandin formation.
- Complement activation.
- Activation of the clotting cascade.
- Formation of leucotrienes, platelet-activating factor and nitric oxide.

What are the pathological effects of all these mechanisms?

- Pyrexia.
- Systemic inflammatory response syndrome (SIRS).
- Shock.
- disseminated intravascular coagulopathy (DIC).
- Multi-organ failure.

Which diseases are mediated by exotoxins?

- Cholera.
- Tetanus.
- Diptheria.

39. Antibiotic Prophylaxis

Define prophylaxis.

Action taken or treatment given to prevent disease.

Aside from antibiotics what other measures can reduce the infective complications of surgery?

- Pre-operative patient optimisation:
  - diabetic control,
  - weight loss,
  - smoking cessation.
- Good surgical technique.
- Good post-operative wound care.

Which patients have particular requirements for prophylaxis?

- Patients with prosthetic heart valves (prevent endocarditis).
- Patients for splenectomy (vulnerable to encapsulated organisms).

How would you classify wounds by risk of infection?

- Clean (<1.5% risk of infection): incision does not break through a hollow viscus.
- Clean-contaminated (<8% risk of infection): viscus other than colon opened.
- Contaminated (15% risk of infection): colorectal surgery and open fractures.
- Dirty (>25% risk of infection): site already contaminated with pus/faeces or a traumatic wound more than 4-hour old.

What prophylactic measures would you advise for each?

- Clean: antiseptic skin preparation.
- Clean-contaminated: single-dose antibiotic.
- Contaminated: broad antibiotic cover, consider short course.
- Dirty: full treatment dose + lavage/debridement.

When might you consider antibiotic prophylaxis in a clean case?

Prosthetic device/material inserted.

Principles of Surgery

PERI-OPERATIVE CARE

THEATRE ISSUES

TRAUMA

ETHICAL ISSUES

1. The Diabetic Patient

How do you assess a diabetic patient in the clinic?

Take a history of the type of diabetic control used, the dosage schedule and the adequacy of control. Particular attention is paid to the propensity to develop hyperglycaemia, ketosis and hypoglycaemia. Ask specifically about the complications of diabetes: nephropathy, sensory and autonomic neuropathy, hypertension, peripheral and coronary arterial disease and retinopathy. The patient looking for these complications is then examined. Look for ongoing infection.

How do you manage the diabetic patient once they are on the ward?

Patients with diabetes often have gastroparesis, and they should fast at least 12 hours before elective surgery. Always try to put the patient first on the list. Patients with diet-controlled diabetes usually just require glucose monitoring. Patients on oral hypoglycaemic agents should have those agents discontinued on the day of surgery. Sulphonyl urea drugs should be withheld at least 1 day before surgery, because of their long half-life. For those on insulin prescribe 5% dextrose with potassium and start sliding scale insulin infusion. Continue the insulin and dextrose infusion until the patient has had a second meal with their normal dose of subcutaneous insulin post-operatively.

What are the potential operative complications in the diabetic patient?

- Infections: diabetics are prone to infection at the surgical site and elsewhere.
- Wound healing: this is impaired in diabetics due in part to microvascular disease.
- Cardiovascular complications: due to macrovascular disease.

2. The Obese Patient

How is obesity classified?

Obesity is classified according to the body mass index (BMI). BMI = weight (kg)/height^2 (m). The normal range is 20–25. Grade I obesity is defined as a BMI 25–30. Grade 2 is defined as BMI 30–40. Grade 3 obesity is defined as BMI >40.

How is obesity associated with excess mortality?

Obesity is associated with excess mortality from diabetes mellitus, heart disease, stroke, pneumonia and accidents.

What are the respiratory complications of obesity?

- Obesity increases the work of ventilation and impairs the function of the chest wall.
- Post-operative atelectasis is more common in obese patients.
- Obese patients may suffer from obstructive sleep apnoea.

What surgical options are there for the treatment of obesity?

Gastric restriction surgery for the severest forms of obesity is an option if other methods have failed.

3. The Hypertensive Patient

What are the surgical causes of hypertension?

- Renal disease: especially renal artery stenosis.
- Coarctation of the aorta.
- Endocrine causes: phaeochromocytoma, Cushing's syndrome, Conn's syndrome.
- Raised intracranial pressure.
- Pre-eclampsia.

A patient in your pre-admission clinic has a blood pressure of 160/100 mmHg. What do you do?

Repeat the blood pressure measurement and enquire about previous recordings to find out if it is just a one-off reading. If it seems likely that the reading is not just a one-off reading look for evidence of end-organ damage: left ventricular hypertrophy, peripheral vascular disease, renal failure and retinal changes (cotton wool spots, macular oedema and haemorrhages). Enquire about a past medical history of myocardial infarction, angina or stroke. The BP should be measured again at least three times with each measurement a week apart. Twenty-four hours ambulatory BP monitoring can be considered. If hypertension is confirmed then liaison is required with the patient's general practitioner (GP) prior to re-scheduling surgery.

What is hypertension is a risk factor for?

Stroke and myocardial infarction. Diastolic blood pressure (DPB) $\geqslant 110$ mmHg is a risk factor for peri-operative cardiac complications. Patients with hypertension have a 25% incidence of either hypotension or an exacerbation of hypertension during the peri-operative period. The risk of peri-operative myocardial infarction is increased if, during surgery, the BP decreases by 50% at any time, or by 33% for 10 minutes or longer.

4. Deep Vein Thrombosis Prophylaxis

Which patients undergoing surgery are at risk of deep vein thromboses ?
- Elderly patients.
- Pregnant patients.
- Patients on the oral contraceptive pill (OCP).
- Patients undergoing orthopaedic or pelvic surgery.
- Patients with malignancy.
- Obese patients.
- Immobile patients.
- Patients with thrombophilia.
- Patients with a previous history of deep vein thrombosis (DVT).

What are the mechanisms of the increased risk?
The mechanisms are classified according to Virchow's triad: increased thrombotic tendency, changes in blood flow and damage to the vein wall.

How do you reduce this risk?
Treat avoidable risk factors: mobilise patients early, use intermittent pneumatic pressure on the legs, use thrombo-embolism deterrent (TED) stockings and use low molecular weight heparin (LMWH).

What are the complications of a DVT?
- Pulmonary embolism.
- Post-phlebitic syndrome.
- Phlegmasia alba dolens.
- Phlegmasia caerulea dolens.

How do you investigate a suspected DVT?
- Laboratory tests: D-dimer estimation is sensitive enough to rule out the diagnosis.
- Imaging: Duplex ultrasound or venography.
- Others: impedance plethysmography, which measures the variations in the volume of calf blood on releasing a blood pressure cuff placed so as to cause temporary thigh venous occlusion.

How do you treat a proven DVT?

Anticoagulate with LMWH and then warfarin for 3–6 months. Thrombolyis may be considered if the DVT is so extensive to cause phlegmasia caerulea dolens. If anticoagulation is contraindicated, then an inferior venacava (IVC) filter may be placed radiologically to prevent pulmonary embolism.

5. Post-operative Complications

How do you classify post-operative complications?

Complications may be local (at the operation site) or general (affecting any other system of the body). They may be classified according to how soon they occur after surgery: immediate – within the first 24 hours, early – within the first 4 weeks and late – >4 weeks post-operatively.

If a patient has a fever post-operatively how would you proceed?

Most patients will develop a transient fever approximately 24–48 hours post-operatively. This is usually attributed to basal atelectasis of the lungs. However, the patient should be fully examined for a source of infection. Particular attention is given to inspecting the wound and examining the respiratory system. Sputum and urine samples can be sent for microscopy and culture. If the temperature is very high, or persistent, then the patient should be examined for further signs of sepsis and blood cultures should be sent to the laboratory.

What are the possible reasons for a patient being hypoxic post-operatively?

- Reduced alveolar ventilation: hypoventilation (airway obstruction, excess opiods), atelectasis, bronchospasm and pneumothorax.
- Decreased diffusion across the alveolar membrane: pneumonia, pulmonary oedema and acute respiratory distress syndrome (ARDS).
- Lack of alveolar perfusion: pulmonary embolus, tension pneumothorax and cardiac failure.

What are the possible reasons for a patient being hypotensive post-operatively?

- Hypovolaemia.
- Cardiac failure.
- Dysrhythmias.

- Effects of medication.
- Spinal or epidural anaesthesia.

6. Imaging Modalities

A patient presents with acute abdominal pain. You suspect perforation or obstruction. What investigations would you request?

A supine abdominal film can establish a diagnosis of obstruction. An erect chest X-ray (CXR) shows free gas under the diaphragm in the case of perforation.

The abdominal film suggests small bowel obstruction. What investigation might you request next and why?

An abdominal computed tomography (CT) scan would confirm the diagnosis. In addition, an abdominal CT may reveal the level cause of obstruction.

The abdominal film suggests large bowel obstruction. What investigation might you request next and why?

A water-soluble contrast enema can confirm the diagnosis and may reveal the level and cause of the obstruction. However, in some cases, interpretation is difficult and a significant obstructing lesion may be missed. CT scanning is valuable for the sick and frail patient, and may be more accurate (and less uncomfortable) than a water-soluble enema.

You suspect a patient has abdominal sepsis. What imaging modalities might be employed and why?

Abdominal ultrasound is particularly useful when there are localising signs. Ultrasound is especially good for assessing the subphrenic and subhepatic spaces, and the pelvis. CT scanning is, however, probably superior. In addition to being able to distinguish between infection and tumours, CT will also allow for biopsy of nodes or masses, and drainage of collections. If there are no localising signs, a radio-labelled white blood cell study may be useful in locating the problem.

A patient has jaundice. What imaging would you use to investigate them?

Abdominal ultrasound will distinguish between obstructive and non-obstructive jaundice. When ultrasound demonstrates obstructive jaundice, further imaging depends on the level of obstruction, the presence or absence of stones in the gall bladder and bile ducts, and the clinical situation. If ultrasound shows duct stones then an endoscopic retrograde cholangiopancreatography (ERCP) can be performed for confirmation and therapy. CT may be useful, particularly if pancreatic cancer is suspected as it can give some indication as to the resectability of the tumour.

Is a plain abdominal film indicated in the investigation of biliary disease?

No, a plain abdominal film only shows about 10% of gallstones. Ultrasound is the investigation of choice for the demonstration or exclusion of gallstones and acute cholecystitis.

A patient has suspected ureteric colic. How do you investigate them?

Unenhanced CT is the technique of choice in suspected ureteric colic. An intravenous urogram (IVU) is a satisfactory alternative. The combination of ultrasound and an abdominal film may be used where radiation/contrast medium are contraindicated, e.g. in pregnancy or in patients with a contrast allergy.

7. Preparation of Patients for Theatre

What needs to be checked before a patient goes to theatre for elective surgery?

The patient should be interviewed and re-examined to ensure that the pathology for which surgery is indicated is still present. It is also imperative to confirm that the patient still wants surgery and to find out if they have any further concerns of queries before going to the theatre. All investigations should be checked (blood, X-rays, etc.) to ensure that they are up to date and that the results are satisfactory. Consent must be obtained from the patient and documented in the notes. Clear instructions should be given to nursing staff regarding administration of medications and fluids pre-operatively. All notes and relevant investigations should accompany the patient to theatre. It is essential to review the medication chart to ensure that there are no medications that are contraindicated with surgery and that any premedications have been prescribed. The surgical team should liaise with the anaesthetics department to ensure that they have made their own assessment of the patient and have discussed the anaesthetic with them.

When are antibiotics prophylactic with surgery?

- Patients with valvular heart disease.
- With implantation of a foreign body.
- Vascular surgery and transplant surgery.
- Amputation of an ischaemic limb.
- Penetrating wounds and open fractures.
- Where there is a high risk of bacterial contamination.

If a patient is already taking on anticoagulants, such as warfarin, what precautions should be taken peri-operatively?

Epidural, spinal and regional blocks are contraindicated. Depending on the indication for anticoagulation, the patient might have to be converted to intravenous (i.v.) heparin (e.g. patients with prosthetic heart valves) or surgery delayed until the course is finished (e.g. first episode of venous thromboembolism).

What precautions should be taken if a patient is on oral contraceptives?

It is recommended that patients stop the OCP 6 weeks before surgery and use an alternative means of contraception.

How do you prepare the bowel prior to elective colorectal surgery?

Put the patient on a low residue diet for 3 days pre-operatively. Twenty-four hours prior to surgery only free fluids are allowed. One sachet of Picolax® may be given in the morning before surgery and a second sachet during the afternoon before surgery.

8. Urinary Retention and Catheters

How can you classify urinary retention?

Urinary retention may be acute, chronic or acute on chronic. Acute retention presents with inability to pass urine, suprapubic pain and mass. Chronic urinary retention presents insidiously with gradual enlargement of the bladder, dribbling incontinence and little or no pain.

What are the causes of urinary retention?

Urinary retention may be caused by local obstruction to urinary flow:

- obstruction in the urethral lumen (e.g. stone or clot);
- obstruction in the urethral wall (e.g. stricture);

- obstruction due to pressure from outwith the urethral wall (e.g. prostatic enlargement or faecal impactment).

Urinary retention may also be due to more systemic general causes:

- post-operatively: due to pain, immobility or medication;
- central nervous system disorders (e.g. multiple sclerosis, spinal tumours);
- medication (e.g. anticholinergics, tricyclic antidepressants).

How do you manage acute urinary retention?

A history should be taken looking especially for prostatism, urinary infection or ureteric colic. The abdomen is examined to confirm the presence of a distended bladder. A digital rectal examination is performed to feel for the prostate, anal tone and perineal sensation. The patient should be catheterised. Further investigations such as urea and electrolytes (U&Es), microbial subluminal univalue (MSU), ultrasonography (US) of renal tract, prostrate specific antigen (PSA) and urethrogram should be considered. Further management will depend on the underlying cause.

What sorts of urinary catheters do you know?

Catheters may be classified according to the material they are made of, e.g. soft latex or silastic (this latter is suitable for long-term use). Catheters may also be classified by size, e.g. the French gauge, where 12 is small and 16 large. In addition, they can be classified according to shape: Foley and Coudé catheters have an angled tip; Teeman catheters have tapered ends.

How do you insert a suprapubic catheter?

Examine the patient to ensure the bladder is distended. Explain the procedure to the patient and obtain their informed consent. Clean the skin over the lower abdomen in the suprapubic region. Infiltrate the skin and down to the bladder with local anaesthetic. Nick the skin with a scalpel. Insert the trocar down vertically above the symphisis pubis. When urine drains back through the trocar, advance the catheter over the trocar and secure it in place.

9. Theatre Design

What are the principal considerations in the design of an operating theatre suite?

- Access: to wards, accident and emergency department, and the sterilisation unit.
- Space: for personnel, storage and equipment.
- Safety standards: air filtration systems.
- Accessory facilities: recovery area, changing rooms and offices.

Where should the operating theatres be located in the hospital?

Theatres should be kept separate from main hospital traffic. They need to be in close proximity to the intensive care unit, surgical wards, accident and emergency, and radiology.

How would you attempt to minimise infection risk in an operating theatre suite design?

The theatre area can be divided into zones: an outer zone containing the theatre reception, which is general access; a limited access zone between the reception and theatres, which includes the corridors and staff rest area; a restricted zone, where only appropriately clothed staff are allowed, such as the anaesthetic room and scrub areas, and an aseptic zone, incorporating the operating theatre itself.

Apart from the operating table, what other services need to be provided for your operating theatre?

- An emergency electricity supply.
- Sufficient power points.
- Wall suction.
- Lighting.
- X-ray viewing boxes.
- Anaesthetic gas scavenging systems.
- An efficient air filtration system with a laminar airflow system.

What accessory facilities would you provide?

- A separate recovery area.
- Changing rooms.
- Washing/toilet areas.
- Staff rest area.
- Offices and seminar rooms.

10. Light Sources in Theatre

What is the main source of light in operating theatres?

The light source is primarily artificial. This can be divided into operative illumination and background illumination.

Why is natural light not used as the main light source?

Natural light is too unpredictable to be used as a main light source, although there is evidence to show that there is a reduction in staff fatigue with natural light.

What factors should be taken into consideration with artificial lights?

Artificial light needs to be of sufficient intensity. This light needs to be focussed and should be under the direct control of the surgeon. The lights also need to be reliable and a back up generator needs to be available if the main lights fail.

Do you know what the light intensity should be approximately?

At the operation site, the light intensity should be about 40,000 lux.

Can you think of any problems associated with artificial lights?

They can create obstacles and affect the characteristics of airflow. They supply heat which increases the temperature in the operating theatre. They are also a source of bacteria so need to be carefully cleaned.

11. Patient Positioning

Why is it important to properly position the patient on the operating table?
- To enable adequate access to the site of operation.
- To prevent injury to the patient.

How may a patient be injured by inappropriate positioning?
- Inappropriate handling may aggravate spinal or joint disorders in a patient.
- Care needs to be taken when positioning the patient's upper limbs, whether by the side or at right angles to the patient as stress may be placed on joints, nerves and ligaments.

What nerves are most likely to be damaged?

Stretching of the arm may lead to brachial plexus injuries. Pole insertion into the canvas sheet may damage the ulnar nerve. Pressure against the leg support bar may damage the common peroneal nerve.

How can the design of the operating table reduce risk of injury?

It is important that patients should be placed on an operating table that moulds to the patients contours to a certain extent. Cushion supports should ensure that the patient should not be in contact with metal structure of the table. Any leg supports on the table should not overstress any joint nor should there be any undue pressure on the patient's lower limbs.

How should a patient be moved to and from the operating table?

Care needs to be taken when moving a patient on or off a table. At least three people should move the patient in a smooth coordinated manner. A slide board should be used to minimise stress. No tubing should be attached to the patient at the time of transfer.

12. Sterilisation

What is the difference between sterilisation and disinfection?

Sterilisation is the process where all viable organisms, including bacterial spores are removed or killed. Disinfection is the process where most but not all viable organisms are removed or killed.

What methods of sterilisation do you know about?

- Heat.
- Irradiation.
- Chemical.
- Filtration.

How can heat be used for sterilisation?

Dry heat achieves sterilisation by oxidising cell components. Glassware can be sterilised at 160–180°C in a hot air oven. Moist heat achieves sterilisation by using saturated steam under pressure. This aids penetration of heat into the material to be sterilisation. To kill bacterial spores, an autoclave cycle of 121°C for 15 minutes or 134°C for 3 minutes is used. Surgical instruments and dressings are sterilised by this method.

How can irradiation be used for sterilisation?

Gamma irradiation energy produces free radicals, which break the bonds within DNA. They can be used to kill spores. Typically, irradiation is used to sterilise small volume items such as catheters, syringes and needles.

What chemical agents are used in sterilisation?

Ethylene oxide can be used to sterilise single use medical equipment such as heart valves. It acts by damaging proteins and nucleic acids.

13. Sutures

Describe the characteristics of an ideal suture material.

- Ease of handling.
- Ease of knotting.
- Ability to "snug down" knots with minimal suture memory.
- Minimal tissue reaction.
- Unfavourable suture surface for bacterial colonisation.
- Provides effective duration of wound support appropriate to the tissue and operation in question.
- High tensile strength.
- Low diameter to minimise tissue damage and scarring.

How do the characteristics of a suture material affect their behaviour?

- Braided suture materials are easier to handle and knot tying is easier. However, the braided surface creates friction and therefore less easy passage through the tissues than monofilament materials.
- Monofilament sutures glide more smoothly through the tissues and incite less tissue reaction, but they are more difficult to knot than braided materials.

How can you classify sutures?

Sutures can be classified according to their source, filament type and absorbability. Sutures can be:

(1) natural or synthetic;
(2) monofilament or multifilament;
(3) absorbable or non-absorbable.

What are the features of natural suture materials?

These sutures handle well and are relatively inexpensive. However, they have unpredictable absorption and can cause tissue reaction and fibrosis. They are absorbed by enzymatic action. Localised infection can occur as they are not monofilament so more likely to trap bacteria. This can lead to wound sinus formation.

What are the features of synthetic suture materials?

Compared to biological sutures, these sutures are inert and absorbed by hydrolysis. They have predictable absorption and strength. However they are more difficult to handle.

Can you tell me the difference between monofilament and multifilament sutures?

Multifilament sutures are strong and handle well. However, they can increase tissue trauma and tend to trap bacteria. Monofilament sutures have smooth surfaces. They do not trap bacteria like multifilaments, but handling and knotting is more difficult.

Can you give me any examples of absorbable sutures and tell me the characteristics of one of them?

- Catgut.
- Polydioxanone (PDS).
- Polyglactin (Vicryl).

Vicryl is an absorbable suture that has predictable strength. It has less tissue reaction and handles well. It may not last long enough for healing when used in some tissues.

Can you do the same with non-absorbable sutures?

- Silk.
- Prolene.
- Nylon.

Prolene is a non-absorbable suture. It is inert and very good for subcuticular sutures. However it is difficult to handle and knot.

What factors involving the suture may lead to wound dehiscence?

- Weak suture material.
- Damage to the suture by a surgical instrument.
- Damage to the suture by diathermy.
- Poor technique in knotting the suture.

When might you use clips instead of sutures?

Staples confer only one advantage in wound closure over sutures: speed of application. Staples are useful when rapid wound closure is desirable or where the wound is large and suture closure would be laborious, e.g. in laparoscopic work.

Describe some suture-needle types and their characteristics.

- Round bodied needle: separates but does not cut tissue, minimal tissue trauma therefore suitable for fragile or delicate tissue.
- Conventional cutting needle: triangular cross section, with the cutting edge on the concave side of the needle. Size 3/0 is adequate for most indications, but for wound closure on the face 4/0 or smaller may be indicated.
- Reverse cutting needle: for tough tissue, triangular cross section, with the cutting edge on the convex side of the needle, which strengthens the needle.
- Atraumatic or blunt needle: used for friable tissue types minimising tissue trauma. Reduced risk of operative needle-stick injury.
- Taper cut needle: provides effective initial tissue penetration, but subsequent protection as the remainder of the needle is round bodied.

14. Retractors

Why would you use retractors in surgery?
Retractors are used in all forms of surgery. They are used to improve the field of vision of the surgeon and protect structures from damage in the surgical field.

What methods of retraction do you know about?
Retraction can be instrumental or non-instrumental. With non-instrumental retraction, the surgical assistant would provide retraction by holding back structures with a swab. This method can be used if the structures are at risk of being damaged by instrumentation. Instrumental retraction may involve self retaining retractors or hand held retractors. Instrumental retractors can also be divided into sharp or blunt retractors.

What hazards of retraction can you think of?
The use of inappropriate retractors or over retraction can lead to organ damage, damage to blood vessels and subsequent ischaemia to the structure it supplies.

Can you tell me about any retractors that you have used in your experience?
A commonly used retractor is the Langenbeck retractor. It is a medium sized retractor that is blunt to avoid damage to the structures it is

retracting. Devers retractors are commonly used in abdominal surgery to provide deep retraction.

When would you use sharp surgical retractors?

These are typically used to retract skin or soft tissues not containing vital structures.

15. Haemostasis

Why is surgical haemostasis important?

- To prevent blood loss.
- To ensure adequate visibility: bleeding obscures the operative field affecting operative technique.
- To prevent formation of haematomas: haematomas may become infected or compress vital structures.
- To reduce the risk of wound breakdown.

What patient factors would affect haemostasis?

- Co-existing medical conditions: bleeding diathesis, chronic liver disease.
- Anticoagulant therapy: heparin, warfarin and aspirin.

What preventative measures can you take prior to surgery?

- Appropriately manage any clotting abnormalities.
- Stop any anticoagulation therapy in sufficient time before the procedure.

How would you ensure adequate haemostasis in theatre?

Good surgical technique: dissection along tissue planes, control bleeding as operation progresses, minimise the area of raw tissue exposed. Use of instruments to control haemostasis: ligation, clips, electrocautery, haemostatic agents (e.g. Surgical), swabs, tourniquets and hypotensive anaesthesia.

Are there any other agents you may use if bleeding cannot be controlled?

- Pharmacological agents (e.g. tranexamic acid).
- Fresh frozen plasma.
- Platelets.

What is surgical diathermy?

Surgical diathermy is a means of applying electrical current at high local current density, to produce a consequent local tissue heating effect. Locally high temperature can be used to produce tissue cutting or haemostatic coagulation.

Is raw mains electricity useful for this role?

No. Diathermy relies upon a high frequency current, typically 400,000–10,000,000 Hz. When concentrated at the tip of a diathermy probe this current produces a local high current density, which exerts locally high temperature, without producing neuromuscular stimulation. Mains electricity operates at a frequency of 50 Hz, which produces neuromuscular stimulation and cardiac dysrhythmia.

What is monopolar diathermy?

In monopolar diathermy current passes from the current generator and through the diathermy probe to the point of tissue application. The locally high current density produces the surgical effect and then returns through the body at relatively lower current density, down a potential gradient to a return plate/diathermy pad and hence to the current generator. The patient's body forms a part of the electrical circuit.

Why does the patient not get a heating effect at the return plate/diathermy pad?

There is a measurable increase in local temperature at the pad, but as the pad is of a relatively high surface area the current density and consequent heating effect is low. Heat generated is conducted away through the tissues and through the circulation.

Why is it a bad idea to use monopolar diathermy on a low diameter extremity such as a finger or penis?

Local current density will be high enough to produce a potential heating effect high enough to cause coagulation within the extremity, causing infarction, severe injury or extremity loss.

Why is it important to avoid placing the return plate/diathermy pad over bony prominences or over operation sites containing metal work when using monopolar diathermy?

These sites are likely to concentrate current and produce local heating and possibly tissue burns. The safest policy is to avoid having internal metal work in the most direct pathway along which current returns to the diathermy pad.

How does cutting diathermy work?

With cutting diathermy the current waveform is that of a continuous sine wave. An electrical arc is struck between the negative electrode and the tissue creating a local heating effect of up to 1000°C, and consequent tissue disruption.

How does coagulation diathermy work?

With coagulation diathermy a pulsed current output, comprising an interrupted sine wave, results in tissue desiccation and a haemostatic coagulation effect.

Why is no return plate/diathermy pad applied to the patient's body when using bipolar diathermy?

With bipolar diathermy the patient's whole body is not a part of the electrical circuit. There is no need for a return plate/diathermy pad as current is applied to and returns from the body via the forceps only. The local heating and hence coagulative effect is exerted upon the held tissues only.

16. Local Anaesthetics

Can you tell me any commonly used local anaesthetics that you have seen used?

- Lidocaine.
- Bupivacaine.
- Prilocaine.
- Cocaine.
- Recently introduced local anaesthetics include ropivacaine and levo-bupivacaine.

How do local anaesthetics work?

They inhibit entry of Na^+ ions though sodium channels in cells with excitable membranes, so blocking an action potential. They are weak bases and are so able to bind to hydrogen ions.

What are the toxic effects of local anaesthetics?

Toxicity arises when the drug is given in overdose or given in the wrong site at the correct dose. The toxic effects of local anaesthetics can be divided into local and systemic effects. Local effects include: inflammatory response (especially esters), neuropathy – if the anaesthetic is injected intraneurally, neurotoxicity – especially high concentrations of lidocaine. Systemic effects include central nervous system depression ranging from perioral paraesthesia to drowsiness, respiratory depression, convulsions and coma. Local anaesthetics also cause cardiovascular effects by interacting with sodium channels on heart muscle. This reduces the force of contraction. They also block calcium and potassium channels. Their action predisposes to hypotension and dysrhythmias.

How would you manage a patient exhibiting toxic effects of a local anaesthetic?

Management is essentially supportive as there is no reversal agent. It is important to assess the airway, breathing and circulation. Stop injecting the local anaesthetic and give the patient oxygen. Be prepared to intubate if necessary. Rapid fluid infusion may be required to help prevent cardiovascular collapse. The patient may require inotropic support. Seek appropriate help.

How does adding adrenaline affect the action of a local anaesthetic?

Adrenaline promotes local vasoconstriction slowing the absorption of the local anaesthetic. The effect of this is to prolong the duration of action of the local anaesthetic and reduce the risk of systemic toxicity. Adrenaline should not be used near terminal arteries such as the fingers and toes, as a reduction in blood flow results in increasing the risk of ischaemia.

How would you calculate the safe maximum dose of a local anaesthetic such as 1% lidocaine?

It is important to consider a number of factors when considering toxicity of a local anaesthetic. These include the site and rate of injection as well as the intrinsic toxicity of the agent itself. One per cent of a local anaesthetic contains 10 mg/ml. The safe dose of lidocaine is 3 mg/kg. In a 70 kg male, a total of 210 mg can be administered. So 21 ml of 1% lidocaine can be safely given.

17. Human Immunodeficiency Virus Patients

What are the high risk groups for human immunodeficiency virus (HIV)?

- Sexually active adults.
- Intravenous (i.v.) drug abusers.
- Patients from endemic areas such as subSaharan Africa.
- Children of human HIV patients.

How can HIV be transmitted from patients to theatre staff?

HIV is a retroviral blood-borne virus. It can be transmitted by needle-stick injury with a hollow needle, contamination of broken skin or by contaminated fluid splashing into mucous membranes or eyes.

What is the risk of transmission?

The risk of transmission following a single percutaneous inoculation is <0.5%.

How would you minimise the risk of transmission?

- Keep cuts and abrasions covered.
- Washing hands before and after patient contact.
- Cleaning hands after contamination.
- Wearing gloves when conducting procedures involving bodily fluids or blood. This also includes changing gloves between patients and washing hands after removal of gloves.
- Avoidance of needle-stick injuries by proper disposal of needles in appropriate containers (needles should not be resheathed).
- Safe surgical practice (e.g. non-handling of needles and double-gloving).
- Ensure spilled fluids are promptly cleaned and that clinical waste is appropriately disposed of.

What steps would you take in the event of exposure to body fluids or blood?

The affected area should be washed with copious amounts of water and encourage open wounds to bleed. The incident should be reported to occupational health for further advice. If out of hours, report the incident to accident and emergency. The incident should be assessed to check the risk of patient/staff member to blood-borne viruses. The source patient may provide a sample which can be tested for hepatitis B and C. With appropriate counselling and consent, the sample can be tested for HIV. A sample is also taken from the affected staff member to be tested in the event that he/she suffers from any symptoms. In high risk contact, post-exposure prophylaxis may be offered. With HIV, this would involve triple therapy.

Should all patients going for surgery be tested for HIV? If not, why not?

No. There are disadvantages to having all patients tested for HIV. All patients require formal consent for the test to occur. Some patients may not agree to have the test performed. A test would cause anxiety to the patient and there are implications of a positive result and all patients would need to be appropriately counselled. There are implications of a false positive test which would be distressing to the patient and a false negative result which would be unduly reassuring. Other factors include the expense of testing all patients, the time taken to conduct the test and how this may delay any treatment.

18. Scoring Systems

What is the purpose of scoring systems?
- Scoring systems provide a way of evaluating the severity of illness, assessing response to treatment and predicting the outcome from various conditions.
- They aid the comparison between patients and units.

What are the characteristics of an ideal scoring system?
It should be validated, easy to use reliable and be able to predict the outcome for specific cases. In the case of the intensive treatment unit (ITU) it should predict the non-survivors for whom admission is futile.

What scoring systems are you aware of?
- Glasgow coma scale (GCS).
- Acute physiology and chronic health evaluation (APACHE).
- Simplified acute physiology score (SAPS).
- Mortality probability models (MPM).
- Revised trauma score (RTS).
- Injury severity score (ISS).
- Abbreviated injury score (AIS).

Briefly describe the GCS.
It gives a score from 3 to 15, with 3 being the worst. It is used to describe the level of consciousness of a patient, and is particularly useful in the management of head injuries. There are three components: motor response scored out of 6, verbal response scored out of 5 and eye response scored out of 4. The best score for each component is always taken, e.g. if a patient has a left hemiparesis but has normal function on the right the motor score would be 6.

Briefly describe the APACHE score.
The APACHE score is made up of the some of three scores – A, B and C.

- A – a score based on acute physiological variables would include rectal temperature, mean arterial pressure, heart rate, respiratory, arterial pH, Na^+, K^+, creatinine, white cell count and GCS.
- B – a score for increasing age.
- C – a score for chronic health by system.

The larger the sum (A + B + C) the poorer the outcome.

When should APACHE scoring be done in the ITU setting?

Within the first 24 hours of admission.

What is the effect of a reduced APACHE score following treatment on outcome?

Despite reduction of the APACHE score with treatment the outcome is unaltered. The initial physiological disturbance is the main determinant of outcome.

19. Wounds

What is the Gustilo and Anderson classification?

The Gustilo and Anderson classification is a classification of open fractures. It is based on the size of the wound and the amount of soft tissue injury. There are three classes in this system.

I   Open fracture + wound <1 cm
II Open fracture + wound >1 cm
III Open fracture + wound with extensive soft tissue, nerve and blood vessel injury

Class III is subdivided into IIIa, IIIb, and IIIc depending on the extent of soft tissue injury and neurovascular compromise.

How can operative ways surgical wounds be classified?

- Operative surgical wounds can also be classified according to the degree of contamination by foreign material.
- Clean: no areas infection encountered during surgery; the alimentary, urinary, biliary and respiratory tracts are not entered; sterile technique maintained throughout the operation.
- Clean-contaminated: clean operation but endogenous flora are encountered; alimentary, urinary, biliary or respiratory tracts are entered under controlled conditions; a minor break in sterile technique may have occurred.
- Contaminated: inflammation seen but without frank pus, alimentary tract entered with spillage of contents, infected biliary or urinary tracts entered, major break in sterile technique.
- Dirty: frank pus found at surgery due to presence of pre-existing infection or prior perforation of a viscus, faecal contamination and retained foreign material in wound.

Can you give some examples of the types of operation that would fit with the classification described in the above question?

- Clean: mastectomy and splenectomy.
- Clean-contaminated: bowel resection with no spillage of contents and transurethral resection of prostate.
- Contaminated: acute appendicitis.
- Dirty: incision and drainage of an abscess and ruptured appendix.

What are the key issues in managing an acute traumatic wound on a limb?

The limb needs to be assessed for fractures and neurovascular damage as these injuries may need to be dealt with formally in theatre. In the absence of any associated injuries to the limb the wound needs to assessed for the need for formal debridement. If the wound is not badly contaminated with foreign material it may simply be washed out thoroughly with saline and closed or dressed. However, if there is obvious contamination then the wound will need to be formally debrided in theatre. An assessment of the patient's tetanus status is also necessary and appropriate cover provided.

What are the general principles of managing chronic wounds?

The main aim is to turn the chronic wound into an acute wound, thereby promoting the formation of granulation tissue and healing. Necrotic material is removed from the wound bed and the wound subjected to regular cleansing and debridement. This will help reduce bacterial load and promote vascularity of the wound bed.

What is the theory behind the use of vacuum dressings in the management of chronic wounds?

The vacuum results in localised hypoxia of the wound bed which stimulates angiogenesis, promotes the formation of granulation tissue and reduces bacterial load.

Can you list some local causes of delayed wound healing?

- Tissue hypoxia.
- Poor blood supply.
- Infection.
- Foreign body.
- Haematoma.

Do you know any systemic causes of delayed wound healing?

- Poor nutrition.
- Anaemia.
- Diabetes.
- Vitamin A and C deficiency.
- Zinc deficiency.
- Glucocorticoid treatment.
- Cytotoxic treatment.
- Jaundice.

20. Tetanus

What organism causes tetanus?

Tetanus is caused by an obligate anaerobic Gram-positive bacillus called *Clostridium tetani*.

Who is susceptible to tetanus?

Those with incomplete immunisation and patients who have not had their 10 year booster. The incidence of tetanus increases with increasing age and in developing countries tetanus has a predilection for neonates.

What are the signs and symptoms of tetanus?

Tetanus has an incubation period of 4–14 days and normally presents with trismus. This is then followed with muscle stiffness, neck rigidity, dysphagia, restlessness and spasms. Reflex spasms can be triggered by small stimuli, these spasms can cause fractures, dislocations and rhabdomyolysis. Sustained facial contraction results in a sneering grin know as risus sardonicus. The back sometimes becomes arched known as opisthotonus. The toxins released have autonomic effects and therefore cause instability of blood pressure, dysrhythmias and cardiac arrest.

What are the names of the toxins released by the tetanus organism?

- Tetanospasmin.
- Tetanolysin.

What is the management of tetanus?

In wounds that may be susceptible to tetanus it is important to perform wound toilet and excise 2 cm of tissue around the wound. If a patient has not been immunised then this should be performed. If the patient has not had a tetanus booster within the past 10 years then this should be administered. If the wound looks tetanus prone then it may be advisable to administer immunoglobulin also.

If generalised tetanus develops, what is the management?
Patients should be admitted to ITU and kept in a quiet environment to reduce tetanic spasms. Most patients will require ventilation. Neuromuscular blocking agents can be used (e.g. vecuronium). Tetanus antitoxin is sometimes administered intrathecally and intramuscularly. Skeletal muscle relaxants (e.g. baclofen) have been used intrathecally with some success, helping to wean patients off diazepam. Antibiotics (e.g. penicillin G) are used against the bacteria but their benefit has not been proven.

21. Dressings

What are the features of an ideal dressing?
An ideal dressing:

1. helps remove excess exudates from the wound,
2. allows for granulation of the wound,
3. keeps the wound warm,
4. protects against secondary infection,
5. is free from particulate or toxic matter,
6. will not traumatise the wound when removed.

Why is excessive exudate a problem in wound healing?
Excessive exudate leads to maceration of both the granulation tissue and the tissue surrounding the wound edge. Exudate is also a site for potential infection. Absorptive dressings remove exudate optimising wound hydration.

What sort of dressing would you use for a necrotic wound?
A moisture donating dressing, e.g. a hydrocolloid containing dressing, which by donating moisture to the wound would help breakdown of necrotic tissue.

What sort of dressing would you use for a granulating wound?
A non-adhesive dressing to preserve granulation tissue. Moisture donating dressings would also be useful.

What sort of bandaging is often used for venous leg ulcers?

Charing Cross four-layer compression bandaging.

What are the four layers of the Charing Cross bandaging system?

Bandage class 3a and 3b with a class 2 support bandage and orthopaedic wool.

What are the potential problems of compression bandages?

They may cause ischaemia due to a tourniquet effect, particularly is used in the presence of peripheral arterial disease.

22. Principles of Fracture Management

What is a fracture and what do its characteristics depend upon?

A fracture is a break in the continuity of a bone. The nature of the fracture is dependent upon the magnitude and direction of the forces causing it.

What are the classical signs of a fracture?

- Tenderness.
- Deformity.
- Swelling.
- Localised raised temperature.
- Abnormal mobility (±crepitus).
- Loss of function (of limb or joint).

What are the immediate management priorities in the management of a fracture?

The principles of Acute Trauma Life Support should be applied. Assess the potentially fractured limbs for the features described above. Specifically examine for, record, and dress any wounds. Record the neurovascular status of the limb. Correct any gross deformities and reduce any fracture-dislocations.

What terms are commonly applied to describe fractures?

- Comminuted: >2 fragments.
- Compound: also known as an open fracture, the surface wound communicates with the fracture.

- Complicated: important soft tissue damage, specifically to nerves, vascular structures or internal organs (all fractures involve some soft tissue damage).
- Transverse: describes the fracture pattern and in these fractures the causative force was usually directly to the site of fracture.
- Spiral: a description of the fracture pattern and how the force was transmitted through the limb (rotational force).
- Greenstick: crumpling of the cortex on the compressed side of the fracture and fracture of the cortex on the opposite side.
- Crush: describes the fracture pattern.
- Avulsion: bony fragment pulled off by traction from a ligament or tendon.

Fractures may be stable or unstable, what does this mean?

Stable fractures are ones in which there is no significant movement, such as impacted fractures, or where the bone ends are held firmly by soft tissues (e.g. periosteum). Unstable fractures are displaced or have the potential to displace. Sometimes reduction may make the fracture stable, although usually some method of holding it reduced is necessary.

What types of fractures may represent emergencies?

- Open fractures: due to the risk of infection particularly chronic osteomyelitis leading to delayed or mal-union. Management involves early aggressive debridement and cleaning which may involve extending the wound. There is some debate over whether primary closure or delayed closure is better. Antibiotics are mandatory and if there is no primary closure then closure should be achieved within 72 hours.
- Fractures with neurovascular compromise: as they may lead to limb ischaemia and/or loss of function. They are treated by early reduction.
- Long bone fractures have a significant association with acute respiratory distress syndrome (ARDS) and so early long bone stabilisation is recommended.
- Fracture dislocations.
- Intracapsular fractured neck of femur in a young patient which should ideally be reduced and fixed within 12 hours.

What reasons are you aware of for fracture reduction?

- Return of function.
- Prevent neurovascular compromise.

- To remove tension from covering soft tissues.
- Removal of impacted soft tissues which will prevent union.

How may reduction be achieved?
- Manipulation.
- Traction: slow reduction, as with cervical spine fracture where manipulation may be too risky.
- Open reduction: very accurate but increased infection risk, particularly if closed reduction failed or if internal fixation required.

What techniques are employed to hold a reduction?
- Plaster casting.
- Fracture bracing.
- Traction.
- Percutaneous fixation with wires or screws.
- Open reduction and internal fixation.
- External fixation.

23. Common Fractures

What common fractures have you come across in your clinical practice?
Fractured neck of femur and Colle's fractures.

Why are they common?
Neck of femur fractures and Colle's fractures are common in older female age groups due to the presence of pathological osteopenic bone. They also share a common mechanism of injury, following falls. Falls are more common in the older age group as they are less independently mobile.

What is the significant decision in neck of femur fractures and what is the most important feature of their management?
Displaced intracapsular fractured neck of femur compromises the blood supply to the head of the femur which leads to avascular necrosis and/or non-union. The decision which must be taken is to whether to preserve or discard the head of the femur in this situation.

How do you describe a classical Colle's fracture?

Transverse fracture of the distal radius, just above the wrist with dorsal displacement of the distal fragment. The resulting deformity of the wrist is commonly described as a "dinner fork" deformity. On X-ray the fracture runs across the radius ~2 cm from the wrist and the ulnar styloid may be broken off. The radial fragment is tilted and shifted dorsally and radially. The distal fragment is also impacted proximally.

What are the complications of a Colles' fracture?

- Mal-union.
- Subluxation of the radio-ulnar joint.
- Tendon rupture: extensor pollicis longus.
- Joint stiffness.
- Sudeck's atrophy.

How is a Colles' fracture different from that which Smith described 20 years later?

A Smith's fracture has anterior (volar) displacement, following a fall on the back of the hand (flexed wrist).

What must be the priority in management of a supracondylar fracture of the humerus?

Exclusion of neurovascular compromise as the brachial artery and any of the 3 nerves (median, ulnar and radial) may be injured. Vascular injury and ischaemia may lead to muscle necrosis and fibrosis.

24. Complications of Fractures

How would you classify the complications of fractures?

Immediate, early/intermediate and late. Within these categories subdivision into local and general is also helpful.

Can you give some examples of each?

Immediate

- Severe haemorrhage (internal and external).
- Internal organ damage, brain, liver, etc.
- Local neurovascular trauma.

Early (Local)
- Skin/soft tissue necrosis.
- Infection and wound break down.
- Loss of alignment and internal fixation failure.
- Gas gangrene and tetanus.
- Compartment syndrome.

Early (General)
- Deep vein thrombosis (DVT)/Pulmonary Embolism (PE).
- Fat embolism.
- Crush syndrome.
- Myositis ossificans.

Late
- Delayed and non-union.
- Failure of internal fixation and fixation device cuts out.
- Joint stiffness and contracture.
- Sudek's atrophy.
- Osteoarthritis.

What are the clinical characteristics of fat embolism?

A clinical triad of symptoms, characteristically respiratory insufficiency, cerebral dysfunction and petechial haemorrhage. Diagnosis made on the basis of the Gurd and Wilson criteria of which the three previous are major criteria.

How do you diagnose problems of union?

Clinically the signs of a fracture persist for longer than expected (>3 months for an adult long bone). These signs are pain, swelling, tenderness and mobility. This is combined with persistent radiological evidence of the fracture.

What is the difference between delayed union and non-union. Where is non-union more common?

Fracture healing progresses by callus formation: this may be visible at 3 weeks or may take longer. There is often much less callus formation with internal fixation. If there is absence of callus with mobility at the fracture site this is indicative of delayed union. Cortication of the fracture ends is strongly indicative of non-union. Non-union is more common with fractures through cortical bone than cancellous bone where there is often impaction.

How is non-union managed?

Non-union may be classified as hypertrophic or atrophic. Atrophic non-union is managed by stimulation of healing through grafting and stabilisation. Hypertrophic non-union will respond to a reduction in mobility through stabilisation. Cancellous bone (from the iliac crest) is used in the majority for grafting as it provides a boney scaffold with living marrow cells which is an ideal osteogenic stimulus. The most fundamental problem in non-union is infection because the infected fracture will not unite until the infection is overcome. Often union may take years or may never occur in which case amputation may be considered.

25. Burns

How would you classify burns in terms of mechanism?
- Thermal.
- Chemical (alkali worse than acid).
- Electrical.
- Radiation.

Burns are usually classified by depth. How is this done?
Clinical evaluation, although definitive results may not be until operative assessment. They are classified as follows:

- Superficial: pink and painful, blistering.
- Deep dermal: pink-white blanching reduced, pinprick sensation impaired/dull.
- Full thickness: black/white, no sensation.

What other features of burns are used to asses their severity?
The total body surface area (TBSA) occupied by the burn. Burns >15% TBSA in an adult are classified as major (>10% TBSA in children). Wallace's rule of 9's is applied: 9% TBSA for the head and each arm, 18% for each leg (front and back 9% each), 36% for the trunk, 1% for the perineum and 1.25% for each hand.

What are the physiological consequences of major burns?
- Hypovolaemic shock: causing reduced cardiac output and increased peripheral vascular resistance.
- Raised metabolic rate.

- Increased haematocrit: plasma lost through the burnt tissue effectively concentrates the blood constituents.
- Cortisol increase: stress response causing catabolism and gluconeogenesis.

What are the key features in the early management burns?

- Intravenous (i.v.) fluid resuscitation: various protocols tailored to the individual patient in terms of burn surface area and time from injury. Fluid regimes must include regular losses in addition to burns losses.
- Airway support: inhalational injury may cause airway compromise due to obstruction by oedema. Tracheostomy may be necessary if there is concern about glottic oedema.
- Escharotomies/fasciotomies: relief of the constricting effect of full thickness burns where tissue ischaemia and necrosis may occur due to tissue damage and swelling negating an already diminished peripheral circulation (due to central hypovolaemic failure).
- Topical dressings; protocols vary, but Flamazine® or non-adherent dressings are usually used.
- The eyes or exposed joints may require early surgery to prevent further damage.

26. Tourniquets

What are the surgical indications for the use of a pneumatic tourniquet?

- To produce an effectively bloodless surgical field, to facilitate anatomy identification and surgical procedure.
- To provide temporary haemostasis in the face of catastrophic uncontrollable blood loss.
- To allow effective regional anaesthesia. For example, Biers block anaesthesia which requires a double tourniquet.

Are there any contraindications to the use of tourniquets?

Crush injury, infection, peripheral vascular disease, sickle cell disease and sickle cell trait are all relative contraindications to the use of a tourniquet.

What size of tourniquet should be used?

The wider the tourniquet the lower the effective pressure required to occlude the arterial circulation. The size of tourniquet can be estimated by the cuff width approximating the diameter of the limb plus 20%.

To what pressure should the tourniquet be inflated?

No consensus opinion exists. The correct answer is as low a pressure as will provide arterial and venous occlusion. One common recommendation is as follows: for the upper limb use a pressure equal to the systolic blood pressure plus 50 mmHg; for the lower limb use a pressure twice the systolic blood pressure.

What are the safe tourniquet ischaemic times?

Again, there is no consensus opinion. The correct answer is as short a time as possible. When using a tourniquet around upper arm or thigh, the surgeon should be informed every half on hour of ischaemic time. Ideally one and a half hours should not be exceeded. The duration of ischaemia should not exceed 2 hours without a reperfusion time of 20 minutes. It should be remembered that such a long ischaemic time will not be safe for all patients particularly in the presence of known relative ischaemia or injury.

What precautions are taken in the application of a tourniquet?

- Neurovascular status should be documented. In the presence of significant peripheral vascular disease tourniquets should be avoided.
- Apply a wool bandage to skin of limb that will lie beneath the tourniquet.
- Apply an appropriate size of tourniquet, securely tied in place, not encroaching the surgical field.
- Exsanguinate the limb by elevation for 2 minutes or expression of blood using an exsanguinating tube. Avoid expressive exsanguination in the presence of tumour, infection or known DVT.

Describe the procedure for application of a tourniquet.

- Timely inflation of the tourniquet to predetermined level, to optimise effective operating time.
- Record inflation pressure and time of inflation.
- During surgery monitor the inflation pressure and ensure the surgeon is regularly informed of the ischaemic time.

Describe the procedure for removal of a tourniquet.

- Request anaesthetist's permission to deflate and remove the tourniquet.

- Record time of deflation.
- Check the neurovascular status of the limb after removal.

Why is it important to request the anaesthetist's permission to remove the tourniquet?

During prolonged ischaemia the products of anaerobic metabolism concentrate in the limb, which is effectively excluded from the general circulation. Upon release of a tourniquet the cardiovascular afterload drops suddenly and a bolus of acidotic, hypercapnic blood is released into the circulation. In a patient with limited cardiac reserve cardiac dysrhythmias and reduced cardiac perfusion may ensue.

Why is it necessary to continuously monitor tourniquet pressure?

Tourniquet pressure drop may allow arterial bleeding obliterating surgical field.

What are the complications of tourniquet usage?

- Pressure neuropathy.
- Tissue ischaemic injury (for example skin necrosis rhabdomyolosis or neuropraxia).
- Vascular endothelial injury and thrombosis.
- Post-operative bleeding. Missed unligated vessels may bleed significantly following deflation.
- Local sickle cell crises may be precipitated by vascular stasis. Tourniquets are relatively contraindicated in the presence of sickle cell disease or trait.
- Tourniquet on lower limb effectively lowers circulatory capacity and increases afterload.

Why may post-operative bleeding be an issue following tourniquet use?

Missed unligated vessels may bleed significantly following tourniquet deflation. Tourniquet deflation and haemostasis prior to wound closure is one way of reducing this risk.

27. Consent

What are the principles of valid consent?
1. Giving of information: the patient must be informed of all the implications of the proposed procedure.
2. Competence: the patient should have the mental capacity to understand these implications.
3. No coercion: the patient must voluntarily agree to have the procedure.

Who is not competent to give consent?
Under the age of 16, children may consent to procedures, but may not withhold their consent. In such cases, consent is required from a parent or guardian. The Mental Health Act (1983) allows for the compulsory treatment of any physical disability or one arising from a mental health disorder, in the case of the mentally incompetent.

Do these precepts always apply?
Emergencies do not alter the patient's rights or the principles of informed consent. However, if it is not possible to obtain consent, e.g. in the case of say a child or an unconscious patient, a clinician may proceed without consent to save life or prevent harm.

Who should obtain consent?
The consultant is responsible for obtaining consent. This task may be delegated, but only to a trained and qualified junior colleague who has sufficient knowledge and understanding of the procedure to ensure that the patient can make an informed decision.

28. Death and Dying

What common symptoms are often seen in a dying patient?
- Pain.
- Urinary incontinence or retention.
- Noisy breathing.
- Restlessness or confusion.
- Dyspnoea.
- Loss of appetite.
- Nausea or vomiting.

What is the analgesic ladder?

When the type of pain has been established (bone, visceral, soft tissue and neuropathic), treatment should follow the World Health Organisation analgesic ladder, with co-analgesics according to the other features contributing to the pain. All patients should start on step 1 of the ladder and should climb up until the pain is controlled. Changing drugs within a step will not achieve an improvement in analgesia. At any step, co-analgesics can be added (e.g. non-steroidal anti-inflammatory drugs (NSAIDs), corticosteroids, antidepressants, anticonvulsants and anxiolytics). It is important to remember to add laxatives and anti-emetics as necessary.

Step 1
- Non-opioids: paracetamol.

Step 2
- Weak opioids: codeine, dihydrocodeine and tramadol.

Step 3
- Strong opioids: morphine, fentanyl, diamorphine and hydromorphone.

How is death diagnosed?

Death is characterised by apnoea, no pulse and no heart sounds, and fixed pupils. If the patient is on a ventilator, death may be diagnosed using the UK brain death criteria: deep coma with absent respirations; the absence of rug intoxication and hypothermia; the absence of hypoglycaemia, acidosis and urea and electrolyte (U&E) imbalance. Diagnosing brainstem death requires the tests to be performed 24 hours apart by two doctors, one of whom should be a consultant.

Which deaths are referred the coroner in England and Wales?

- Unknown cause of death.
- The patient was not seen by a certifying doctor within 14 days of death.
- Death was caused by medical treatment.
- Death was suspicious.
- Death occurred within 24 hours of admission to hospital.
- Death was caused by a road traffic accident, an industrial disease or accident, a domestic accident, violence, neglect, abortion, suicide or poisoning.
- Death occurred during legal custody.
- Where there is any claim for negligence against medical or nursing staff.
- Death of a foster child, patient under the Mental Health Act (1983), mental defectives or service pensioners.

Notes

Notes

Notes

Notes